Mind & Muscle

Blair Whitmarsh, PhD

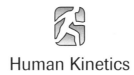

Human Kinetics

Library of Congress Cataloging-in-Publication Data

Whitmarsh, Blair, 1966-
   Mind & muscle / by Blair Whitmarsh
     p. cm.
   Includes index.
   ISBN 0-7360-3753-5
   1. Bodybuilding--Psychological aspects. 2. Physical fitness--Psychological aspects. I.
Title: Mind & muscle. II. Title.

   GV546.5 .W48 2001
   646.7'5--dc21   00-054270

ISBN: 0-7360-3753-5
Copyright © 2001 by Blair Whitmarsh

Developmental Editor: Cassandra Mitchell; **Assistant Editors:** Wendy McLaughlin and Dan Brachtesende; **Copyeditor:** D.K. Bihler; **Proofreader:** Kathy Bennett; **Indexer:** Sharon Duffy; **Permission Manager:** Toni Harte; **Graphic Designer:** Nancy Rasmus; **Graphic Artist:** Tara Welsch; **Photo Manager:** Clark Brooks; **Cover Designer:** Keith Blomberg; **Photographer (cover):** Tom Roberts; **Art Manager:** Craig Newsom; **Illustrator:** Tom Roberts; **Printer:** Bang Printing

Human Kinetics books are available at special discounts for bulk purchase. Special editions or book excerpts can also be created to specification. For details, contact the Special Sales Manager at Human Kinetics.

Printed in the United States of America   10 9 8 7 6 5 4 3 2 1

Human Kinetics
Web site: www.humankinetics.com

United States: Human Kinetics, P.O. Box 5076, Champaign, IL 61825-5076
800-747-4457
e-mail: humank@hkusa.com

Canada: Human Kinetics, 475 Devonshire Road Unit 100, Windsor, ON N8Y 2L5
800-465-7301 (in Canada only)
e-mail: orders@hkcanada.com

Europe: Human Kinetics, Units C2/C3 Wira Business Park, West Park Ring Road,
Leeds LS16 6EB, United Kingdom
+44 (0) 113 278 1708
e-mail: hk@hkeurope.com

Australia: Human Kinetics, 57A Price Avenue, Lower Mitcham, South Australia 5062
08 8277 1555
e-mail: liahka@senet.com.au

New Zealand: Human Kinetics, P.O. Box 105-231, Auckland Central
09-523-3462
e-mail: hkp@ihug.co.nz

This book is dedicated to the memory of my first training partner: my dad, Garfield Garnet Whitmarsh. He bought me my first set of weights when I was 14 years old and woke up early in the morning to "train" with me. I will never forget his willingness to spend time doing the things I enjoyed, even when they were not his interests. He was a wonderful, loving father who always encouraged me and told me that I could do anything I desired. I am eternally grateful for the love, patience, instruction, and mentoring he so willingly gave. I loved him very much and will never forget him.

CONTENTS

ACKNOWLEDGMENTS

In 1979, I picked up the latest edition of *Muscle Builder* magazine and saw a great picture of Robbie Robinson on the cover. I was so impressed with his "ice cream scoop" biceps that, even though I was the stereotypical 98-pound "weakling," I was convinced that health, fitness, and strength training would become an important part of my life. Not until I attended graduate school, however, did I begin to appreciate the relationship between mind and body and its effect on fitness and muscular development.

Unsure of what the final product would look like, I began to write this book a little at a time. Along the way, many people have shared their time, advice, and insight, and for that I am extremely grateful.

First, I would like to extend a special thanks to my immediate family. My wife, Lorraine, was a tremendous support and encouragement through the challenges of writing this book. Her words of wisdom and understanding were invaluable. I believe this accomplishment is as much hers as it is mine. My children, Karina, Jolayne, and Tana, and Skipper the dog give me great joy and provided me with the motivation to pursue my dreams. My mom, June Whitmarsh, has given me unconditional love and continual encouragement. She took a keen interest in this book and was a wonderful sounding board. My sister and her husband, Renai and Atticus Harivel, kept me on track by continually asking me, "When are you going to finish that book?" I am grateful to have such a wonderful family, and I love each of them very much.

My photographer, John Yanyshyn from Visions West Photography in Victoria, British Columbia, was the most understanding and professional photographer I have worked with. His previous experience with bodybuilding, both as a competitor and a photographer, was a considerable asset. I welcomed his creative flair as he went far beyond the call of duty, helping to find appropriate models and working with each image until it had the aesthetic appeal I was looking for. I also appreciate the models, Kevin Psaila, Marnie Fargo, Tomi Zdrilic, Melissa Connell, Johnny Olarte, Jodi Michaels, Brad Nault, Leslie Michaels, Kevin Lathangue, and Blair Watling, for their enthusiasm during the photo shoots and willingness to have their photos included in this book.

There are others who played a significant role in the completion of this book and who deserve recognition: Rebecca Lloyd, Andrew Heming, Bill Luke, Lena Johannesen, Beth Horn, Victor Konovalov, Dan Wagman, Mike Bodner, Gina Masoni, Carol Semple-Marzetta, and Neal Hamilton for their unique contributions to each chapter sidebar; Denise Unrau, for her invaluable editing work in the early stages of the manuscript; and Heidi Paa, for her willingness to write the chapter for women and cowrite the chapter on competition, and for her insightful comments on the rest of the book.

Finally, I would like to extend gratitude to my publisher and editor. Ted Miller believed in me enough to ask me to write this book for Human Kinetics. He treated me with respect, and his professionalism was much appreciated. Cassandra Mitchell patiently and expertly shepherded the manuscript through the process of becoming a book, offered creative ideas and provided valuable input that made the process smooth and enjoyable.

CREDITS

Tables and Exercises

Tips for Improving Motivation adapted from Waitley, D. 1987, *The psychology of winning.* (Chicago: Nightingale-Conant).

Tables 4.3 and 4.4 are adapted from *Hormonal manipulations* ©William N. Taylor, by permission of McFarland & Company, Inc., Box 611, Jefferson NC 28640. **www.mcfarlandpub.com.**

Table 8.1 is adapted, by permission, from Thomas R. Baechle and Roger W. Earle, 2000 *Essentials of strength training and conditioning*, (Champaign, IL: Human Kinetics) chapter 22.

Focusing guidelines for bodybuilders adapted, by permission, from John Hogg, 1995 *Mental skills for swim coaches*, (Edmonton, Canada: Sport Excel Publishing) 7.38.

Black Box Visualization is adapted from J. Syer and C. Connolly, 1984 from *Sporting body sporting mind*, (Cambridge, MA: Cambridge Publishing Company).

Exercise 11.1 is adapted from Mark H. Anshel, *Sport Psychology* 3rd ed., © 1997 by Allyn & Bacon. Adapted by permission.

Figures

Figure 6.1 is adapted from M.E.P. Seligman, 1990. *Learned optimism,* (New York: Alfred A. Knopf).

Figure 8.3 is adapted, by permission, from Thomas R. Baechle and Roger W. Earle, 2000 *Essentials of strength training and conditioning*, (Champaign, IL: Human Kinetics) chapter 22.

Photos

John Yanyshyn, photographer, except where otherwise noted. Photos on pages 82, 85, 90, 97, 106, 123, 201, 220, 232, and 240 by Tom Roberts.

©Action Images 154

©Joe Giblin/Newscom.com 279

Darnell Dedrick ©Richard A. Goodman 126

Moses Ajala ©Richard A. Goodman 134, 175

Darvin Hinkle ©Richard A. Goodman 270

Harold Phillips ©Richard A Goodman 264

©iphotonews.com/Brooks 171

©Dennis Light/Light Photographic 261

©Chuck Mason/International Stock 53

©Nova Stock/International Stock 252

©Robert Randall/International Stock 209

CHAPTER 1

Checking Your Readiness for Success

You may be wondering if this book is for you. You are interested in health and would love to have a lean, muscular physique, but you have never considered yourself a true bodybuilder. In other words, no one is going to mistake you for a brick wall on the beach or ask you to quit blocking the sun.

The bodybuilders you see in muscle magazines are huge, ripped, and unable to buy clothes at "regular" stores. They are not "regular" men and women interested in fitness. While it is true that some people choose to make a career out of shaping and toning their bodies to perfection, most of the people you see in gyms and fitness clubs are not professional bodybuilders. They may want a change in overall body shape and health, be consistent in their training patterns, use nutritional supplements, and have a strong muscular appearance, but they have neither the time nor the desire to be professional bodybuilders. Bodybuilding is no different from any other sport: many people play hockey, basketball, and tennis, but only a few compete at the professional level.

Any person interested in changing his or her body shape through weight training, aerobic exercise, good nutrition, and proper rest is a bodybuilder. Whether you are at the beginning stages of shaping your body or have been a highly competitive bodybuilder for years, you are still a bodybuilder. *Mind & Muscle* is written primarily for those who understand the basic principles of weight training, have basic knowledge of nutrition, and have been working out regularly for at least one year.

You see, the desire to look a certain way and to present an acceptable body image to those around you is not uncommon. Nor is it a new phenomenon. Throughout the ages, people have been concerned with the way they present themselves to others. In ancient Greece, athletes were revered—in fact, they were often elevated to the status of "god"—for their physical strength, power, and endurance. Murals, pottery, sculpture, and other artwork of ancient Greece are evidence of the fascination its people had with the muscular, athletic, and naked human body.

Of course, not every culture gives as much attention to the development of the human body as did the Greeks. In the days of the Roman Empire, for example, personal fitness or body image was not important. It was a culture of decadence and self-gratification, and it was characterized by the love of "spectator" sport. In fact, those who participated in sport were usually of lower socioeconomic status or were so-called criminals. Again, this is evident in ancient Roman art, in which the human body was usually depicted fully clothed in nonathletic scenes of self-importance.

Ancient or modern, every culture has had something to say about the importance of the human body. In contemporary society, the human body has once again taken a front seat. We have come full circle, adopting many of the philosophical attitudes held by the ancient Greeks about the human body, but with one significant addition: the desire for a level of fitness that promotes overall health. So while the preferred body presentation of contemporary society is one of strength and muscular tone, it is also with an overriding concern for health and wellness.

Sure, bodybuilding is about sculpting an attractive physique, but it is much more. Today much of body development is invisible to the human eye: cardiovascular fitness, aerobic and anaerobic capacity, quality of life, absence of disease, and longevity. It is this sense of body wholeness that the bodybuilding lifestyle is all about. If you are serious about becoming a bodybuilder, you must also be serious about cardiovascular fitness, muscular endurance and strength, flexibility, body composition, and the absence of disease. What good is an attractive body if it is falling apart on the inside?

Bodybuilding: A Mainstream Lifestyle

You do not have to look far to see how bodybuilding has influenced contemporary culture. From the Hollywood actor wanting to "beef up" for a movie role to the high school athlete getting ready for the big game, bodybuilding has clearly moved to the forefront. In today's world, the term *bodybuilder* is a term of acceptability, but it has not always been this way.

From the late 1800s until the 1930s, bodybuilding was not a popular activity. With the exception of Eugen Sandow, born in 1867 in what is now Germany, who was the first bodybuilder, those who did engage in it were seen as egotistical "freaks." It was not until the 1940s, when Joe Weider published *Your Physique*, a weightlifting instructional magazine, that bodybuilding would begin the long road to mainstream acceptance. By 1965, Joe and Ben Weider had changed the name of *Your Physique* to *Muscle Builder,* created the Mr. Olympia contest (in which winners are now awarded a bronze statue of Sandow), and developed an educational approach to the sport of bodybuilding. With the help of Arnold Schwarzenegger, and the release of *Pumping Iron* in 1977, the Weiders began to transform bodybuilding from a "cult" activity to an integral part of the mainstream lifestyle.

The pinnacle of current acceptance came on January 31, 1998, when the International Olympic Committee's (IOC) executive board granted the International Federation of BodyBuilders (IFBB) recognition as a federation. From then on, it seems, bodybuilding has been grounded in the mainstream. Indeed, it has become an integral part of the lifestyle of competitive athletes, actors, dancers, musicians, and others. But bodybuilding is more than a sport. Its most important contribution is not just to the sporting community but also to society as a whole. Over the past 52 years, Ben Weider has been convincing people that bodybuilding is not simply a sport but a lifestyle. In his message to the IFBB following the IOC decision, Ben stated "bodybuilding is important for nation building,"and with 170 countries making up the IFBB family it becomes clear why.[1]

The Mental Side of Bodybuilding

Psychological dimensions of individual and group behavior are becoming increasingly important and obvious in competitive sport, whether it be amateur or professional. Athletes and coaches are beginning to realize that the major difference between winning and losing is psychological in nature. How many times have you heard a post-game interview during which an athlete on the winning team maintains that victory was the product of wanting it badly enough, or wanting it more than the other team?

Most sport psychologists believe that within every athlete exists a genetically determined physical limit on his or her athletic potential—a potential few athletes ever reach. What separates superior athletes from good athletes is mental preparation and attitude during training and competition.

The foci of mental training are mental performance, physical ability, and preparation. Sport psychology is not just for the "head cases," or for people who need a "shrink." Most people who use mental-training strategies view themselves not as sick but as healthy, goal-directed athletes who want to improve their skills to a higher level of performance.

Whether recreational or elite, a bodybuilder requires an advanced level of strength, flexibility, balance, muscular symmetry, and body coordination. It takes commitment and a strong desire to succeed for those attributes to be developed, and it is for this reason that personal trainers, strength and conditioning specialists, and bodybuilders spend many hours developing training programs, working out, and preparing meals. As mentioned earlier, bodybuilding is more than working out or trying to eat right. Bodybuilding is a healthy lifestyle that takes dedication to get the best results. Therefore, it is not enough for a bodybuilder to just develop and improve physical and technical skills, it is equally important for a bodybuilder to have a training program that includes a systematic and structured plan for mental skill acquisition. Serious bodybuilders, committed to muscular size, ripped definition, and symmetrical enhancement, must include mental training in their bodybuilding program. Think of sport psychology as another component of training—a set of tools designed to make the best athlete possible. A mental skills program will help you focus on improving those things that you already do well and identifying the skills you have yet to acquire.

Sport psychology is not magic or instantaneous. To develop the best body possible, you will need to be mentally prepared for almost every workout, and certainly for every competition. You will need to learn, develop, and practice specific psychological techniques such as

- short- and long-term goal setting,
- positive thinking and affirmation,
- performance profiling,
- motivational strategies,
- relaxation and complete breathing,
- arousal- and attention-control techniques,
- self-coaching, and
- mental rehearsal and visualization.

Many coaches and athletes maintain that peak performance is somewhere between 40 and 90 percent mental. While it is impossible to know the exact extent to which mental factors affect athletic performance, it is clear that the mind plays a significant role.

You must treat mental training the same way you treat your physical training, nutritional regimen, and sleep habits. Would you enter a bodybuilding contest without working out in the gym months earlier? Could you have developed that ripped physique by adhering closely to a high-fat, low-protein diet? Obviously, the answer is no. Every bodybuilder knows that a ripped, muscular body takes a strong commitment to lifting weights and adhering to a sound nutritional program. The commitment to developing mental skills is just as crucial.

You can develop mental skills by practicing them in a diligent and consistent manner, just as you lift weights, eat soundly, get enough rest, and take nutritional supplements. For mental skills to be effective, you must practice them every day.

State of Mind

As a bodybuilder, have you ever blamed other people for a poor workout or a lack of body definition? Have you ever made statements like "If she would only give me more help as a spotter, then I could get in a couple more reps," or "if my spouse would cook more low-fat food then I would have those six-pack abs that I want." Have you blamed a poor performance solely on yourself? Do you ever talk to yourself with negative statements like "it does not matter that the gym has lousy equipment; I should be much bigger than I am."

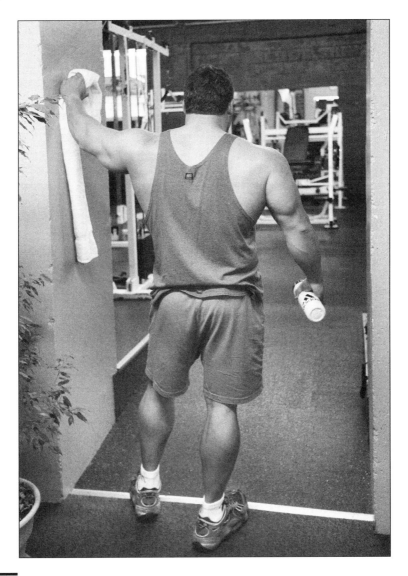

Approaching each workout with a positive frame of mind is the first step to bodybuilding success.

Of course, you are not responsible for a gym's lack of equipment. You are, however, responsible for your state of mind during a workout. You are also responsible for your level of readiness and for your attitude, negative or positive, as you enter the gym. For example, you can think of your workouts as a necessary evil to get the body you want, or you can view them as an opportunity, even a challenge. Bodybuilders who yearn for the end of each workout will clearly get less out it, and will most likely end early by skipping critical sets and completing fewer reps. If you view training as a challenge, however, you will savor each set and rep, feeling pride with each improvement. Sooner or later, you will likely find that you will be disappointed if you cannot complete a workout.

Most successful bodybuilders enjoy training and competition. They love their sport, have fun doing it, and are motivated by the challenge. They understand the importance of frame of mind, knowing that the attitude they bring to the gym or stage will enhance or hinder their performance.

As a bodybuilder, you are responsible for your performance as well as the body you develop. If you take the time to prepare mentally for training and competition, form your goals, learn to focus your attention, and take control of your own destiny, you will succeed, in some cases far beyond your expectations. You will see yourself as successful, regardless of the outcome, and will experience the feeling of accomplishment that accompanies peak performance.

As the saying goes, "You are what you eat." Obviously, a strong commitment to sound nutrition is essential if you want to build a strong and ripped physique. What may not be so obvious is that what you think about can have a dramatic impact on your performance. In fact, your mind-set has more influence on your body than does nutrition. If you do not have the mental fortitude to stick with your workout program, eat appropriate muscle-building foods, and get sufficient rest, you will never build the body you want. In other words, negative attitudes, negative expectations, and negative behaviors will ultimately lead to diminished body development (see figure 1.1). Conversely, positive attitudes, positive expectations, and positive behaviors will inevitably lead to enhanced body development. Perhaps a more appropriate saying for the athlete: "You do what you think."

More Than Just Another Book!

This is not simply a book that applies psychological principles of sport to the world of bodybuilding. This is an interactive book that will assist you in developing the mental outlook and skills necessary to succeed as a bodybuilder. The psychological principles and techniques presented in this book have been utilized extensively with athletes from a wide range of sports, including bodybuilding. Along with valuable information to think about, each chapter in *Mind & Muscle* presents different skills exercises. Complete each exercise as directed, and remember to practice these skills consistently and often. This format enables systematic and controlled development of mental skills. When you complete this book, you will have learned the necessary mental skills to be a successful bodybuilder and can then begin to apply them to your training. This book outlines a mental skills program to supplement an existing physical training and nutritional regimen.

As a bodybuilder, your potential is substantial, probably greater than you allow yourself to imagine. The true mark of a champion is the ability to realize that potential and to perform accordingly. Developing the mental skills necessary for optimal muscle development will go a long way in helping you realize your potential. But the self-knowledge and self-worth that result will help you achieve your potential in many other areas of your life.

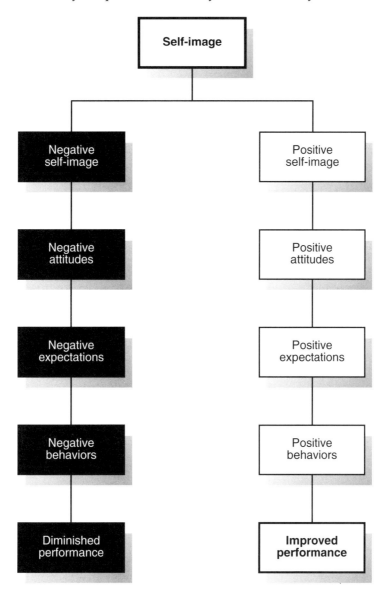

Figure. 1.1 Positive and negative self-image.

Psychological Skills for Bodybuilding

There is no shortage of good information about the benefits of strength training. You have more than 600 muscles in your body, and they are all competing for your attention. They want to become stronger, larger, and more shapely. Every decade after the age of 30, people lose muscle fiber at a rate of 3 to 5 percent. That means, without a bodybuilding program, as much as 30 percent of muscle fiber is lost by the age of 60! Moreover, as muscle size and strength decrease, weight gain and obesity can occur. With an increase in muscle fiber, however, the basal metabolic rate increases. Adding just 1 pound of muscle to your frame will increase your caloric demands by approximately 50 calories per day.

Virtually every study on strength training has found that it plays a significant role in many health factors, including bone mineral density, percentage of body fat, glucose metabolism, and blood pressure. Studies also show that resistance training may contribute to better balance, coordination, and agility. Bodybuilding is a lifestyle of muscle growth, nutrition, proper rest, and the interplay between the emotional, physical, and mental components of human life. It is a lifestyle that is concerned not only with fitness and shaping the human body but also with vitality in play, work, and relationships.

Certainly, bodybuilding will improve your outlook on life and help you overcome various challenges. To get the most enjoyment and success from pumping iron, however, you will need to have a specific set of psychological skills: personal responsibility, assertiveness, personal confidence, a deep commitment to goals, the development of a process-oriented outlook on life, and self-awareness. These skills are hierarchical; that is, each one builds upon the other. Strength in one builds strength in the others.

For example, if you take personal responsibility for your own workouts and body shape then you will eventually experience a take-charge attitude. This attitude translates into becoming more assertive in your environment and making gains in self-confidence. You will learn to believe that you can be successful in everything you attempt. Eventually, as you embark on your own bodybuilding journey, you will find that, more than your sculpted body, you will most appreciate the process you had to go through to achieve it. You see, like on-the-job training, the skills necessary for effective bodybuilding are also the benefits that one gets from bodybuilding.

Personal Responsibility

In general, people do not like to accept personal responsibility for their actions, particularly if their actions have negative consequences. As a bodybuilder, however, you must monitor your own weight-training program, nutritional practices, sleep patterns, and personal motivation levels. No one else can do it for you. You will never get those hard-packed muscles

The Commitment to Strength and Fitness: Rebecca J. Lloyd

Rebecca J. Lloyd, BSc, MA, is the Director of Personal Training at The Fitness Group where she overseas client care and quality fitness programming, supervises personal trainers, instructs group fitness, and makes numerous presentations. Her areas of specialty include sport psychology and chore-ography for sport aerobics, women's fitness, and the training of figure skating competitors. In 1994 she finished fourth at the 1994 National Sport Aerobics Competition. Her academic achievements include the publication of her masters thesis in *The Sport Psychologist* and acceptance into the Simon Fraser, PhD program. She provides her thoughts below about making a commitment toward the goal of strength and fitness development:

Training the body for 'optimal physique' takes 100 percent commitment. When you are getting ready for competition, you don't have a general idea of what you need to do, you have a specific plan for every step of training. Success in fitness and bodybuilding is 99 percent preparation and 1 percent luck. It takes a full year to optimally periodize physical, mental and routine training. If you are ready to take the plunge, I recommend that you find an experienced trainer, surround yourself with supportive friends, find motiva-tional pictures, look forward to your planned "cheat meals," and enjoy your journey.

In 1994, I began to consult with fitness competitors. I admired the chiseled physique they achieved because of their commitment to training. Soon I found myself intrigued with the whole preparation process. I decided to experience the training for physique and fitness firsthand. For a year, I relied on an experienced trainer, recorded every weight training exercise, followed a nutrition regimen, and worked with a gymnastics coach. My focus paid off when I won the 1999 fitness title for Ottawa.

Ongoing communication with my trainer and trust in my program were the keys for staying on track. I loved sharing my achievements, such as my new gymnastic skills and increasing the amount of weight I could lift. Lifting weights was my favorite part of preparation since I experienced inner and outer strength development. I found it to be a meditative experience. The only thing on my mind when I was lifting was channeling my muscular exertion.

Recently, I've been training a novice regional competitor. Seeing her compete last weekend brought back many happy memories of my own competitive experience as well as all the athletes I've been fortunate enough to meet. Whether they were national champions or first time participants, each athlete I worked with had an exhilarating competitive experience. From what I've seen over the years, I'm inclined to believe that winning is internal, because winning is a state of mind. Just walking on stage makes you a winner.

If you have never competed, I urge you to watch a fitness show. Seek out a mentor to help you get started. If you've been competing, continue to train to be your best and the winning will take care of itself.

if you do not spend time in the gym, eat right, and get adequate rest. The good news is, the personal responsibility you develop in bodybuilding will transfer to the rest of your life. You will begin to take control of all that you do.

Assertiveness

Assertiveness training is now commonplace across North America. Indeed, it has become a multimillion-dollar business. Just look at a daily newspaper and you will probably see an advertisement for an assertiveness-training course. Being assertive includes standing up for your rights and for things that are important to you.

Assertiveness is required of the bodybuilder and is a natural byproduct of the bodybuilding lifestyle. Assertive athletes are intense, confident, and persistent. They continually challenge themselves to reach optimal performance. As a result, many bodybuilders often report that weight training has helped them to overcome their shyness, although it was not their intention.

If you want to have ripped abdominals or massive arms, you must give it all you've got during your workouts. You will need to challenge yourself in the same way that a lifting partner or coach would challenge you. You will find that you have no choice but to develop an assertive quality to get the most out of your workouts.

Like standing up for yourself produces self-confidence, assertiveness in bodybuilding creates positive self- and body esteem. *Body esteem* is a narrowly applied term which refers to the way that you feel about your external body appearance. Numerous studies have found that self-esteem and body esteem were higher in study participants involved in weight training than in those not involved in weight training. Moreover, people who are most satisfied with their bodies tend to be more assertive in all life situations. This is due, in part, to significant improvements in body composition, strength, and endurance. Albert Bandura, a world-renowned psychologist, believes that people with high self-esteem take more personal control over a wide variety of situations and behaviors outside the world of sport and physical activity. Clearly, body esteem is a critical component of self-esteem and plays a significant role in how people see themselves.

Personal Confidence

To realize your goals as a bodybuilder, to achieve muscular strength and gain size, you must believe that you are capable of achieving those goals. Personal confidence is developed over a period of years, and is the direct result of effective thinking and continued success. Julie Ratzlaff, fitness trainer at Trinity Western University, has found that people who lift weights enjoy a greater level of self-confidence than those who do not lift. According to Ratzlaff, this is primarily a result of learning to set goals and overcoming the physical challenges involved in weightlifting.

The physical effort necessary for bodybuilding creates the belief that you can do anything if you put your mind to it. The consistent experience of overcoming physical challenges, and then seeing significant changes in body size and shape, results in positive thinking patterns. When practiced consistently, positive thinking becomes automatic and natural, and leads to repeated successes. This, in turn, leads to greater self-confidence. Confident bodybuilders think they can, and they do!

Commitment

Anyone involved in pumping iron knows that if you want the results, you must be disciplined. You work out four to six times per week, eat four to six carefully planned meals each day, take nutritional supplements and vita-mins religiously, and make sure that you are in bed early so that you can get adequate rest before your morning workout.

Few athletes are able to reach the level of excellence without personal commitment. They know that they only hurt themselves by deciding to skip workouts or not follow their diets for extended periods of time. There is no room for cheating in bodybuilding! Indeed, bodybuilding is no different from other aspects of life: if you fail, it is most often due to a lack of commitment and discipline.

A Process-Oriented Outlook

We live in a "fast food" age, and with it comes a "fast food" mentality. We do not want to wait for anything if we do not have to. For a bodybuilder, however, waiting is a fact of life. The process that a bodybuilder must go through is long and requires patience. Improved muscle mass and shape do not happen overnight. In fact, significant gains in bodybuilding can take years. Thus, your level of commitment will be one of the most important universal skills you will develop.

Patti, a friend and new fitness participant, was so frustrated that she had not seen significant fat loss after six weeks of running that she contemplated quitting. "It wasn't working anyway," she said. It was not until a fitness trainer persuaded Patti to enjoy the process and let the results take care of themselves that she agreed to continue on with her exercise program.

Experienced bodybuilders know that physical change in the muscles requires adequate time and great physical effort. Few find the road to bodybuilding success to be smooth. In fact, it is their ability to stay focused and committed to health and fitness over a period of many years that has made them the bodybuilders they are.

As you grow as a bodybuilder, both in size and experience, you will begin to enjoy the process. No doubt you have goals that you want to accomplish such as losing 40 pounds of fat, gaining 2 inches on your biceps, and/or increasing your bench press by 100 pounds. These goals may all be attainable goals, but each one will take time and no one knows exactly what that time

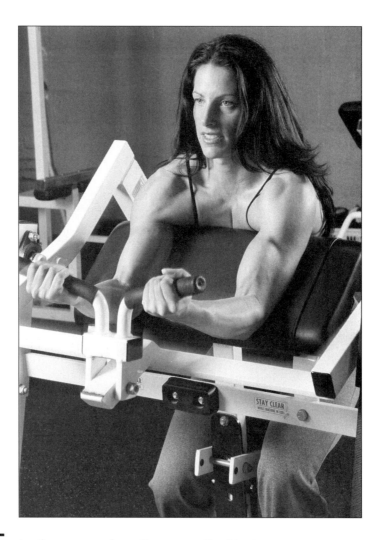

Learn to enjoy the process of creating your optimal body.

will be. The process of being continually challenged and seeing your body transformed before your very eyes is every bit as rewarding as reaching the goals themselves. In fact, experienced bodybuilders will often comment that the process is more rewarding. Your body will change, but if you expect change to occur overnight you will be disappointed.

Physical Identity

Physical identity is a critical component of the mental skill required in bodybuilding. Conflict between your perceived self, real self, and ideal self may lead to counterproductive behaviors. Your perceived self refers to how you think of yourself right now, the real self is the person that you really are, and the ideal self is the plan that you have for yourself "down the road." For example, suppose you are dissatisfied with your biceps and, considering them a weakness rather than a strength, try to minimize showing them at competitions. Your ideal self as a bodybuilder includes having biceps that are peaked and separated from the main part of your upper arm. Although your training partner, fellow gym mates, and competitors know that you have a great set of biceps (real self), you see yourself as having inadequate biceps (perceived self). In this situation, you would need to improve your physical identity.

Faulty physical identity can also occur in the opposite direction. In this situation, you perceive yourself to have reached or exceeded your ideal self when, in fact, everyone else knows that your real self has a long way to go to reach the ideal. This scenario is usually manifested by bodybuilders who see no need to commit to their training programs. After all, they are already better than everyone else. It also seems to be these bodybuilders that have the most difficulty accepting poor scores at competitions. Even though all spectators and officials believe that they have been treated fairly, they still believe they have been mistreated.

Having a healthy physical identity in bodybuilding means knowing who you are so that you can develop your full potential. In developing your physical identity, it is helpful to take on the role of a coach or training partner, trying to observe yourself through his or her eyes and assessing how he or she sees you. While this is important in bodybuilding, it is equally important in life. By developing a healthy physical identity, you will have developed the tools necessary for solving many of your own problems, because you will truly know yourself. Physical identity makes all other psychological skills easier to learn and master. In fact, physical identity is the basis for most of the applied mental skills (i.e., goal setting, relaxation, visualization, concentration, and confidence) that you will be learning later in this book.

Are You Ready to Be a Bodybuilder?

To improve your body, you must know exactly what aspects of your body need improvement. What are your strengths and how can you enhance them? What are your weaknesses and how can you overcome them?

You can determine your strengths and weaknesses in a variety of ways. One of the most obvious methods is to ask your training partner to observe you working out or posing and then provide feedback on your personal strengths and weaknesses. Likewise, you can obtain feedback from a close friend, spouse, or family member about your bodybuilding attributes.

While such opinions and observations are objective, useful, and valuable, ultimately you will need to determine and acknowledge your own strengths and weaknesses. I have never seen a good bodybuilding gym that is not covered in mirrors, and I have never seen a successful bodybuilder who does not use them to compare him- or herself to other bodybuilders. The mirrors not only help you evaluate your strengths but also give you an idea of what you must do to improve your body and minimize your weaknesses on stage.

While mirrors are primarily for perfecting lifting form and posing routines, they can also help you see how you are developing in the three critical areas of size, symmetry, and definition. These three areas are what bodybuilding judges will be looking at when comparing one bodybuilder against another. They are also the body attributes that are most noticed by bystanders while you are at the beach, pool, or just going for a run in your tank top. To be recognized as an elite bodybuilder, you must be able to show that you have a body that is both muscular and pleasing to the eye. A balanced, symmetrical body, whether you compare upper to lower, back to front, or side to side, and little body fat will make it easy for you to show off your hard work.

As a bodybuilder, you must begin to evaluate yourself on four major areas: muscular development, nutritional habits, lifestyle patterns, and mental skills. Muscular development is the development of your muscular frame, including the size of various muscle groups, body symmetry, strength, flexibility, and power. Nutritional habits are the ways you eat and prepare food, as well as what you eat and drink, including fats, carbohydrates, proteins, supplements, and sport drinks. Lifestyle patterns are those aspects of your lifestyle that may affect body development, such as sleeping patterns, use of recreational drugs and alcohol, and social activities. Mental skills, which as we already know are crucial to achieving peak performance,

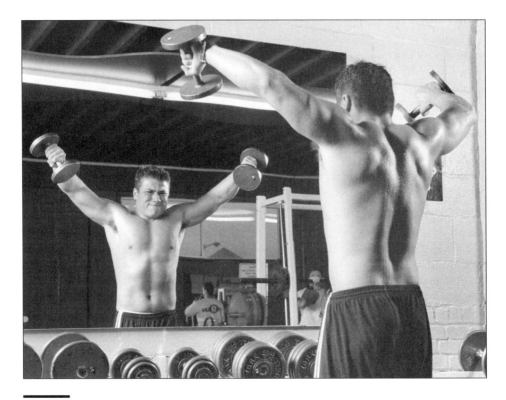

Working out in front of a mirror helps you perfect form and visually evaluate your strengths and weaknesses.

include the skills that we have already mentioned in this chapter and those such as relaxation, visualization, concentration, and self-coaching which will be discussed in later chapters.

For each of the four major bodybuilding areas, you will need to generate a list of attributes essential to developing the ultimate body. Then rate yourself on each attribute. It is important that you be completely honest with yourself. Information is only valuable if it is accurate. It is also important that you reevaluate yourself on a regular basis for comparison and to measure your progress.

The following four exercises will assist you in becoming more aware of your bodybuilding strengths and weaknesses. The self-awareness you gain by completing these exercises now will be useful in subsequent chapters, where you will learn to adjust your attitude, set goals, and create action steps for goal accomplishment. *(It is a good idea to photocopy these pages before writing on them so that you can use them again in the future.)*

Exercise 1.1 will assist you in determining which attributes you need to develop the optimal body. You may find that brainstorming with fellow bodybuilders is the most effective way to complete this exercise.

In preparation for more specific profiling exercises, exercise 1.2 will help you to reflect on your personal attributes and determine your strengths and weaknesses. You might want to use some of the attributes you came up with in exercise 1.1.

Exercise 1.3 is a more specific profiling exercise designed to help you assess your muscular development, nutritional habits, lifestyle patterns, and mental skills. An example of a finished profile is provided. It is important that you read all the instructions before proceeding. *(Be sure to photocopy exercise 1.3 as you will need to fill out one profile for each of the four skill development areas.)*

The final profile exercise, 1.4, is specifically designed for competitive bodybuilders.

You understand what it takes to be a bodybuilder. Spend some time evaluating your own strengths and weaknesses. Then you will be ready to move on and you'll know that you can accomplish almost anything if you are willing to put your heart, mind, and time into it. Bodybuilding is no different. Bodybuilding, as a lifestyle and a competitive sport, focuses on creating a body that satisfies you, in terms of fitness and health, as well as image. To create the best opportunity for achieving that body, you will have to learn to use the power of your mind more effectively.

You simply cannot take your mind for granted. Your physical identity goes a long way in determining whether or not you will succeed as a bodybuilder and mental attributes such as being committed and having a process-orientated outlook are essential. For example, it may be easy to plan an exercise program but it is not nearly as easy to stay motivated. As you go through this book, remember that bodybuilding has as much to do with mental development as it does with physical development.

Exercise 1.1 Attributes Required for Bodybuilders

Instructions: List attributes that may be required of a bodybuilder under each heading. An example is provided for each heading to get you started.

	Muscular development	Nutritional habits
1.	Strong, powerful pecs	Eating a low-fat diet
2.		
3.		
4.		
5.		
6.		
7.		
8.		
9.		
10.		

	Lifestyle patterns	Mental skills
1.	Getting adequate sleep	Focus in the weight room
2.		
3.		
4.		
5.		
6.		
7.		
8.		
9.		
10.		

Exercise 1.2 Personal Evaluation

Instructions: Briefly describe your strengths and weaknesses as a bodybuilder.

Muscular development strengths	Muscular development weaknesses
Nutritional habits strengths	**Nutritional habits weaknesses**
Lifestyle patterns strengths	**Lifestyle patterns weaknesses**
Mental skill strengths	**Mental skill weaknesses**

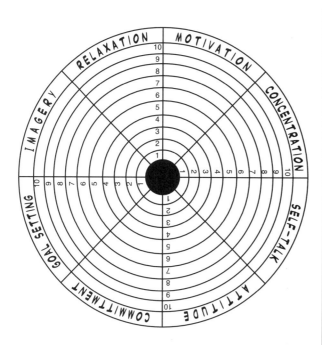

Mental skills	
Attribute	Rating
1. Motivation	5
2. Goal setting	8
3. Desire	
4. Intensity	
5. Concentration	4
6. Relaxation	6
7. Imagery	5
8. Self-talk	3
9. Dedication	
10. Attitude	2
11. Commitment	2
12. Arousal control	

Instructions

1. Make copies of this table and use it to assess twelve attributes of muscle development, nutritional habits, lifestyle patterns, and mental skills. Write the twelve attributes in the table above.

2. Identify the eight attributes that you consider the most important for creating the optimal body. Note: They may or may not be your current strengths.

3. Write these eight attributes in the outer ring of the profile wheel.

4. Rate the eight attributes (from 1 to 10) based on your ability to perform them. To assist you with the rating, use the following scale:

    1=terrible   3=poor   5=adequate   7=good   9=outstanding
    2=very poor   4=mediocre   6=fine   8=excellent   10=superior

5. With a colored marker, color the arc that corresponds to your rating for each attribute. This is a graphical representation of your mental skills attributes.

6. Repeat this exercise every two to three months to assess your development.

Exercise 1.3 | Self-Awareness and Ratings in Bodybuilding

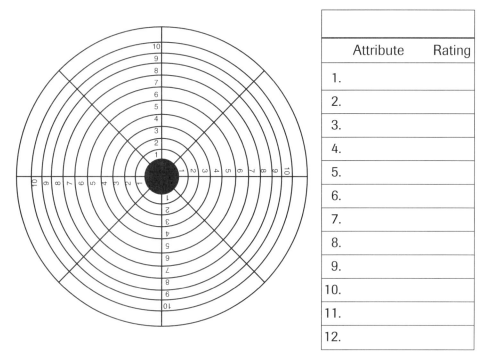

Attribute	Rating
1.	
2.	
3.	
4.	
5.	
6.	
7.	
8.	
9.	
10.	
11.	
12.	

Instructions

1. Make copies of this table and use it to assess twelve attributes of muscle development, nutritional habits, lifestyle patterns, and mental skills. Write the twelve attributes in the table above.

2. Identify the eight attributes that you consider the most important for creating the optimal body. Note: They may or may not be your current strengths.

3. Write these eight attributes in the outer ring of the profile wheel.

4. Rate the eight attributes (from 1 to 10) based on your ability to perform them. To assist you with the rating, use the following scale:

1=terrible	3=poor	5=adequate	7=good	9=outstanding
2=very poor	4=mediocre	6=fine	8=excellent	10=superior

5. With a colored marker, color the arc that corresponds to your rating for each attribute. This is a graphical representation of your mental skills attributes.

6. Repeat this exercise every two to three months to assess your development.

Exercise 1.4   Competitive Experience Profile

Instructions: Think about each of the attributes listed below and, using the rating scale from exercise 1.3, rate yourself on each attribute, first assessing your best performance and then your performance last month.

Preparation

	Best performance	Last month		Best performance	Last month
Dedication			Training session(s)		
Commitment		¿	Motivation		
Effort			Staleness		
Goal accomplishment			Sleeping pattern(s)		
Nutritional habits			Training partner		

Competition

Concentration			Desire to succeed		
Confidence			Anxiety		
Nervousness			Stage presence		
Muscular definition			Choreography		
Muscular size			Audience appreciation		

Mental skills

Imagery			Motivation		
Relaxation			Energizing		
Self-talk			Arousal control		

CHAPTER 2

Constructing a More Powerful Physical Identity

We live in a culture that is fascinated by the human body. In fact, historical overviews on the cultural understanding and interpretation of the human body indicate that human civilization has always had a strong focus on the way the mind and body link. Whether it be the separation of mind and body, as was the case with Plato, Aristotle, and Descartes and the concept of dualism, or the intertwining of mind and body in Eastern philosophy, the body has been center stage.

Contemporary society and Western culture is probably more fascinated with the human body than any society or culture before us. The difference being that the current fascination is not with the anatomical or physiological function of the body but with the way the body looks. In other words, people in Western culture tend to be more concerned with the external health of the body than with internal health or the way the body functions.

Beauty Is in the Eye of the Beholder

As is evident in the myriad historical and cultural differences in beauty ideals and practices, definitions of beauty are culturally bound. While many societies consider body shape and size important determinants of beauty, societies differ on which body shape and size is attractive. In some cultures, such as in Polynesia and some parts of Africa, rotund men and women are considered attractive, because rotundness is associated with prosperity, prestige, and wealth. In other cultures, particularly Western cultures, slimmer body shapes for women and sleek, muscular body shapes for men are generally considered most attractive. This is not to say that different "ideal" body types are not favored in some circles. For example, an emaciated look for women (e.g., fashion runway models) is considered ideal for some, while a well-shaped muscular physique on a woman is considered attractive for others. For men, muscular definition is important, but thinness can also be important depending upon the situation and societal circle. While large is better among male bodybuilders, many in the mainstream do not consider bulky muscles attractive. The reality is that even though the majority of Western culture prefers a slimmer body shape for women and a muscular body shape for men it is clear that beauty is truly in the eye of the beholder.

Of course, the current Western "ideal" of male and female beauty has not always been the case. Although the concern for physical appearance in men is a relatively recent phenomenon, there is a strong tradition of body concern for females. In the latter part of the 19th century, the voluptuous woman was fashionable. A plump body was encouraged for reasons of both health and beauty. This ideal began to change in the early 20th century when, before World War I, the slender "Gibson Girl" grew into vogue. A small waist as well as a large bust and hips being ideal, the corset and padded undergarments became quite popular. After World War I, as flat-chested flappers replaced the curvy ideal, women removed their padding and let out their waistlines. Beauty was seen in cosmetically decorated faces and the near absence of female secondary sexual characteristics, and women used various strategies such as starvation diets in an attempt to reduce body weight.

With the onset of the depression, the narrow waist returned, and female secondary sexual characteristics such as wider hips and larger breasts were back in fashion, as typified by such actresses as Mae West and Greta Garbo. By the 1940s and well into the 1950s, the voluptuous woman once again became the ideal. As Marilyn Monroe burst onto the scene, women's legs, hemmed stockings, and high heels became the focal points of beauty. The onset of the skinny, non-curvy shape in the 1960s, popularized by the fashion model Twiggy, was the last major shift in the Western beauty ideal. While the emaciated waif was popular for a brief time in the late 1980s and early 1990s, and the athletic look has recently been more popular, the overall look of a thin, not-too-curvy shape has remained the Western ideal for women. Based on the look of most of today's fashion models, this trend is going to continue in the 21st century.

Males and females differ in their perception of the ideal body. In modern Western society, females tend to prefer the thin, ectomorphic physique while males tend to prefer the muscular, mesomorphic physique. The ectomorphic physique is identified as a body that is slim with both low body fat and little presence of muscle tone. The mesomorphic physique is one that is largely muscled with low levels of body fat. Once again, not everyone will agree with the body "ideals" held up by society, but more often than not, society upholds values that are generally agreed upon by most of its individual citizens. While there is not doubt that the increase in bodybuilding among women is changing the notion of the ideal female body upheld by society, it is likely that women will continue to identify thinner figures as ideal.

There is some evidence that the notion of an ideal body shape is formed early. A 1993 study published in *The Journal of the American College of Nutrition* found that adolescent girls tended to see themselves as fat and wanted to lose weight, even when they were at or below normal weight. Adolescent boys, on the other hand, were more likely to view themselves as being too small, wanting to gain weight. As for specific body parts, although girls were more likely to want larger breasts, most of those studied wanted smaller thighs, buttocks, and hips. The boys wanted a bigger, more muscular appearance with bigger upper arms, chest, and shoulders, and smaller buttocks and waist.[1]

Obviously, bodybuilding can play a significant role in attaining the ideal body. More important, bodybuilding can have an impact on body image and self-esteem.

Self-Esteem and Body Image

Self-esteem describes the way a person feels about himself or herself. Typically an expression of approval or disapproval, self-esteem can be expressed in voice, posture, gesture, or performance. A multidimensional concept, self-esteem encompasses many different factors, including social, emotional, academic, and physical self-concept.

Body image has been defined as "a person's mental picture of his or her body, oftentimes in relation to an external standard." Body image can be thought of as a person's perception of the cultural standards for attractiveness, the extent to which one's self-evaluation matches this standard, and the perception of the relative importance of this match by the individual and cultural group. Like self-esteem, body image is a multidimensional construct with many contributing physical factors. Kenneth Fox, a well-known psychologist in the area of self-esteem and body image, has suggested that physical self-worth (body image) is a significant factor in overall self-esteem and includes four significant factors: sport competence, attractive body, physical strength, and physical condition.[2]

Clearly, bodybuilding has a direct role to play in the development of three of those factors, namely, attractive body, physical strength, and physical condition. Developing a muscular, strong physique does much more than fill your clothes. A strong, fit, and attractive body leads to a better body image and ultimately to greater confidence and self-esteem. It is difficult to find an activity that can have as dramatic an impact on overall self-esteem as bodybuilding.

Interestingly enough, the link between body image and self-esteem varies between males and females. Females tend to place more importance on their

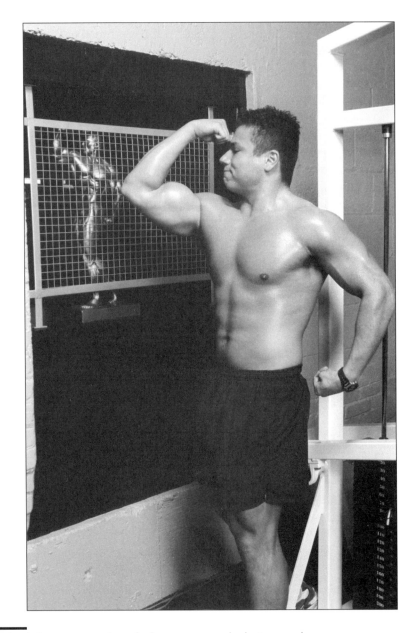

Your body is an expression of who you are and what you value.

physical appearance than do males. According to the *Nebraska Symposium on Motivation*, "whereas men primarily view their bodies as actively functional, as tools that need to be in shape and ready for use, women primarily see their bodies as commodities, their physical appearance serving as an interpersonal currency."[3] Indeed, women tend to use body weight and shape as the prime indicators of physical attractiveness, whereas men tend to rely on upper body appearance and strength as their cues of attractiveness. Again, in addition to all the other tremendous benefits of bodybuilding—improved cardiovascular function, better flexibility, and enhanced quality of life, to name a few—male or female, there is simply no better activity to improve body image than bodybuilding and fitness training.

Body Image and Bodybuilding

When you get up in the morning and head to the bathroom, what is one of the first things you do? If you are like most people, you look in the mirror. Although you may be satisfied with many aspects of your body, you may have a few body features you are less than satisfied with. Whether you think you are overweight, have short legs, are too hairy, or need larger muscles, most likely you will be able to find something about your body that you would like to change. Indeed, more people begin an exercise program to change their bodies than for health reasons.

It is not that the health benefits of bodybuilding are impossible or unimportant. As already discussed, few activities can provide as many health benefits as bodybuilding. Rather, it is that people cannot see health. Health is a concept. It is experienced; it is felt internally. Most people are interested only in what they can see. That means, they are keenly aware of how they look, particularly in comparison with others, and they know what their ideal body is. Unless you're under strict medical direction or supervision, looking good in a new bikini, losing 5 pounds, and fitting into clothes are stronger motivators for exercise than are its many health benefits. The good news is that there is nothing wrong with being motivated to improve your body, as long as that motivation is kept in check.

Psychological Benefits of Bodybuilding

Besides the myriad physical benefits of bodybuilding, there are many psychological benefits as well. One weight trainer, Bob, found that bodybuilding increased his energy level and his ability to cope with life, and stabilized his moods. Bob had exercised inconsistently for many years, but he finally decided to make a serious commitment to bodybuilding two years ago. Before that commitment, Bob maintained a consistent weight of 200 pounds and a body fat percentage of about 14 percent. He was tired all the time and lacked the energy to get through the day. Since committing to bodybuilding and following a nutritious diet, however, he has been sleeping better and enjoying a significant increase in energy. He has even improved his endurance in intense training sessions. While his body weight has held steady at around 200 pounds, his body fat percentage has dropped to 9 percent.

Can bodybuilding play a significant role in helping you feel better about yourself, relate better to other people, effectively manage stress, increase your confidence, and change your emotional stability? You bet! Bodybuilding provides many psychological benefits, including enhanced emotional well-being, reduction of anxiety and depression, increased self-confidence and energy, and an improved ability to cope with stress.

Enhanced Mood

Physical fitness is positively associated with mood. This is evidenced by the fact that as people improve physical fitness, they tend to experience a corresponding increase in the quality and quantity of positive mood levels. Mood, one aspect of emotional well-being, is considered a temporary state of emotional or affective arousal. Mood changes have been studied in a variety of exercise settings, including strength training and such forms of aerobic exercise as running, swimming, and cycling. While participation in aerobic activities seems to have the greatest impact on overall mood levels, strength training has also been shown to have an effect on stabilizing positive mood levels.

Reduced Anxiety and Depression

Every person has experienced an anxious situation, certainly. For many, dealing with particular people or life events produces anxiety. This type of anxiety, *state anxiety*, is a temporary form of apprehension that varies in intensity depending upon the strength of the anxiety-producing cause. For a small segment of the population, however, anxiety can be a stymieing force that affects all behavior and relationships. This type of anxiety, *trait anxiety*, is characterized by continual apprehension no matter the context of the anxiety-producing cause. Those with trait anxiety find everything from speaking in public to playing a musical instrument to be anxiety-producing. Trait anxiety accounts for 30 percent of total hospitalization and 10 percent of all medical costs.

Exercise, including bodybuilding, can have a positive effect on both state and trait anxiety. In fact, anxiety can be diminished significantly depending on whether it is experienced as somatic anxiety (characterized by increased heart and breathing rates, perspiration, and "butterflies") or cognitive anxiety (characterized by mental anguish, worry, and concern). Even a single exercise session can reduce somatic anxiety and the reduction can last for as much as six hours after exercise. A regular exercise program, of at least two exercise sessions per week for at least four months, can have a similar effect on both state and trait anxiety, with the reduction in anxiety lasting as long as 15 weeks after exercise has stopped. While research, to this point, is unable to show that exercise can cause a significant reduction in cognitive anxiety, it remains clear that intense exercise can have a dramatic effect on state anxiety.

As much as 25 percent of the North American population suffers from mild to moderate depression. As the number of people with depression increases, so does the number of people who rely on mood-altering drugs and alcohol, antidepressants, and counseling. Studies have shown that exercise is effective in treating mild to moderate depressive disorders. In fact, in some cases, aerobic exercise is just as effective as therapy, for the simple reason that exercise has an antidepressive effect. While most of the research has focused on aerobic exercise, a few studies have targeted anaerobic exercise, finding that anaerobic exercise reduces mild to moderate depression as effectively as aerobic exercise.

Increased Self-Confidence

As already noted, improving your body image through a well-designed program of weight training and aerobic exercise will have a positive impact on your self-confidence. Self-confidence, a component of self-esteem, is a global term that describes your level of confidence in a variety of situations. When you are self-confident, you will believe that you are capable of doing almost anything whether it be making a financial decision, athletic activity, or the ability to mix in a social situation. In a report submitted to the Canadian Fitness and Lifestyle Research Institute, 58 to 74 percent of the research studies conducted between 1980 and 1994 reported positive changes in self-esteem among subjects involved in exercise programs. The changes in self-esteem lead to improved self-confidence, which translates into the ability to meet people, form lasting relationships, engage in mastery attempts, and commit to a healthy lifestyle.[4]

Increased Energy and Ability to Cope

Work, spouse, kids, errands, chores, appointments, "to do" lists, traffic—everyday stressors can wear you down, sapping your energy and leading to burnout at an early age. Indeed, if you are as busy as most people these days, making time to exercise could seem impossible. The good news is, as your fitness level increases, so does your energy! People who exercise not only have more energy and vigor, they recover from strenuous exercise more quickly than non-exercisers, and they experience fewer feelings of emotional and physical burnout in the gym, home, and workplace.

One of the more interesting stress-related psychological constructs to come to the forefront in the last few years is that of hardiness, which is a quality that enables you to withstand or cope with stressful situations. Hardy people, like bodybuilders, have a sense of personal control over external events and a deep level of commitment and purpose in daily life. While bodybuilding and a hardy personality can both have an impact on stress-related illness, it is the combination of the two that best protects your health over the long term.

So, if being fit brings with it a decrease in fatigue, depression, and tension, it only makes sense that you would want to maintain a high level of fitness for the rest of your life. Adding 20 pounds of hard-packed muscle, getting ripped, looking good on the beach—no matter what your reason for becoming a bodybuilder, instituting a solid nutrition and strength-training program is beneficial for both your physical and emotional long-term health.

Three Personality Traits Essential to Bodybuilding

The term *personality* is difficult to define. Its meanings range from "character" and "the measure of social effectiveness" (a person may be viewed as having a great personality, a terrible personality, or no personality at all) to highly technical definitions employing mathematical formulations. For the most part, *personality* refers to whatever it is that makes a person a person, that is, who they are, what they do, and how they act. When a person is said to have done something "out of character," that judgment is based on prior knowledge of the person's personality.

What does personality have to do with bodybuilding? Personality plays a significant role in your motivation for strength training, including goals you set and your ability to handle plateaus in training or defeats in competition. Not everyone will be able to excel in bodybuilding, just as not everyone will excel in team sport, music, drama, or academic study. It is personality that directs people into different life activities and personality that drives people to be successful in their chosen pursuits. For the bodybuilder, there are three aspects of personality that are crucial for success: positive attitude, motivation, and emotional intelligence.

Positive Attitude

Attitudes are simply habits of the mind. The patterns of thought you develop about particular situations and events eventually become ingrained attitudes about those situations and events. In sport, athletes have attitudes about themselves, other people, and their environments. These attitudes are based on training, instruction, and experience. While some of your attitudes, namely, the positive attitudes, enhance your ability to function successfully, other attitudes, the negative attitudes, impair your ability to function at an optimal level.

A student of mine, Brad, could always find something wrong with the gyms he trained in. Some were too small, another played bad music, and another was simply too busy. As time went on, Brad became less motivated to work out. There was always something that did not meet his standards, and eventually Brad stopped working out altogether. He let his negative attitude about the training environment affect him to such a degree that he quit training. If only Brad had adjusted his attitude before his attitude adjusted him.

The Wanting and Wishing of Motivation: Andrew Heming

Andrew Heming, BHK, CSCS, is a personal trainer at Fitness World and a part-time instructor at Trinity Western University in Langley, Canada. He also is a consultant with Performance Master Consultants, a Langley-based company that trains strength and conditioning professionals. He shares some of his experiences below:

As a personal fitness trainer, I group people into one of two categories: wishers and wanters. Wishers are dreamers who would like to look like bodybuilders or fitness models, but that is as far as they go. Wishers use phrases like, "if only . . .," "I just can't seem to . . .," and "I sure would like . . . ." They may have good intentions, but good intentions mean nothing without action. If wishers are unwilling to get off the couch and go to the gym, eat properly, or get the rest they need, no matter how much they wish it, they will never develop their dream physique.

A former client, Alison, was a great wisher. I put her on a program that would help her "tone up," but no matter how committed she was, she never seemed to lose weight. She was frustrated almost to the point of tears. At first, I thought I made a mistake with the program until I found out that Alison was eating a lot of junk food. I advised her to cut back on her alcohol consumption, stop eating doughnuts at work, and log her nutrition. As much as Alison wished to get lean, she was just not willing to make the necessary changes.

Wanters are different from wishers. They know what it takes to make physique changes and are willing to do it. Wanters use phrases like, "I will . . .," "I can . . .," and "I am going to . . . ." Wanters know that the secret to making a positive change to their physique is making positive changes to their whole lifestyle.

Another client, Ryan, a wanter, came to me with a goal to lose fat and gain muscle. Ryan realized that I could not make him lean or make him gain mass, but I could give him the tools and the information he needed to achieve his goals. Ryan took responsibility for his own body and took it upon himself to carry out the program I designed. It has been over 18 months, and Ryan is still training and improving his physique.

You cannot stand still. Everything you do either moves you closer or farther away from your goals. Your success in changing your physique will depend more on what you do with your life than what you do in the gym. Train to stimulate muscle growth, eat to fuel your body, and sleep to enhance recovery and growth, and you will turn your dreams into reality. In short, be a wanter, not a wisher.

Steps in Changing Attitudes

Attitudes are not always easy to change. The purpose of attitude-adjustment exercises is to evaluate your current attitudes and change those that are counterproductive. Your attitudes play a critical role in your behavior. Negative attitudes are damaging and need to be replaced with positive, productive attitudes. As successful bodybuilders know, "you do what you think."

There are five steps in creating a change of attitude.

1. Recognize. Before you can change your attitudes, you must first identify what those attitudes are, both positive and negative. Are you satisfied with the amount of time you spend in the gym? Do you enjoy eating a low-fat diet? What do you think about your training partner or other bodybuilding competitors? For each of these questions, you have formed an attitude that will either help or hinder your bodybuilding future.

2. Accept. Once you have determined your existing attitudes, positive or negative, you must then accept that these attitudes truly represent what you think. You may discover that one of your prevailing attitudes is not a true representation of who you are. You may also find that you are not completely comfortable with some of your attitudes, but if you wish to change them, you must learn to accept them as true and accurate.

3. Evaluate. After recognizing and accepting your attitudes, you can begin to evaluate them and determine which ones need adjustment. Your training partner, spouse, and other significant people in your life can play a key role in assisting you with this step. They can help you identify which attitudes are counterproductive to your bodybuilding goals.

Because many attitudes are interdependent, you will need to evaluate each attitude independently. For example, a negative attitude about your training may be directly related to a negative attitude about your gym. You may hate to train there because it has no natural light and it feels stuffy. You would first need to change your attitude about the gym (or move to another gym). Then your attitude toward training would be easier to change. Part of this step is identifying and prioritizing your counterproductive attitudes so that you can adjust the most debilitating ones first.

4. Adjust. Now it is time to reform those attitudes that need adjustment. The attitudes could be about your progress, your body, your potential, your training partner, your gym, or other aspects of your bodybuilding program. There are many ways to change counterproductive attitudes such as using positive affirmations or conducting a reality check. These strategies along with others are explained in more detail later in this chapter.

5. Integrate. Once you have adjusted a counterproductive attitude, you will find that you feel more comfortable with your bodybuilding program. Now you can start to integrate your new attitudes into your existing

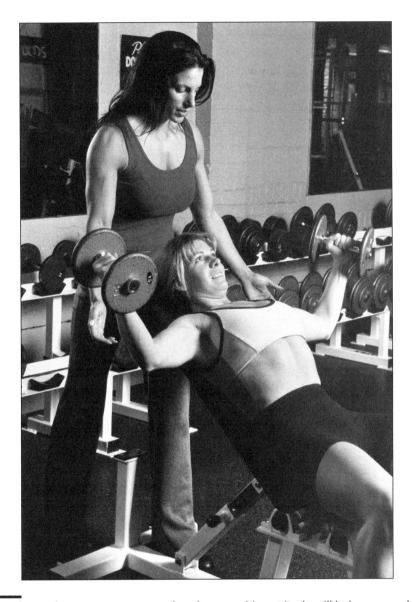

During the workout you must remember that a positive attitude will help you reach your goals.

attitudes about bodybuilding. This can be accomplished simply by stopping your negative thoughts and replacing them with a positive response. For more specific information on ways to integrate your new attitudes into your bodybuilding lifestyle continue reading to the end of this chapter. Then you can begin to take control of your new attitude by applying it in appropriate situations. By enforcing your new, positive attitudes in this way, positive thinking will become as ingrained as your old, negative attitudes once were. Eventually, your old attitudes will completely disappear.

Identifying Your Attitudes

The following exercises are designed to help you identify and evaluate your attitudes about certain aspects of the bodybuilding lifestyle. As noted earlier, identifying your attitudes is the first step toward making necessary adjustments. Every bodybuilder wants to accomplish as much as possible. It would simply be foolish to let a nonproductive attitude stand in the way. Read each task and think about it carefully before you start writing. Be honest. It is important that you identify your personal attitudes, not those that sound nice or that others want to hear.

Exercise 2.1 Examining Your Attitudes

Task 1: Describe how you currently see yourself as a bodybuilder. Use simple words (e.g., strong, ripped, weakling, soft, etc.).

Task 2: Describe how you currently view yourself as a bodybuilder, focusing only on the positive. Rephrase negative descriptions in positive terms. For example, "I am a small and weak bodybuilder" should be rephrased as "I will get bigger and stronger with more commitment to my training."

Task 3: Identify your current attitudes about each category listed below. Positive or negative, your attitudes should be clear and honest.

Training

Diet

(continued)

Training partners

Personal trainer

Sport science (i.e., sport psychologist, physiologist, nutritionist, physiotherapist, massage therapist)

Training gym

Competitors

Competition venues

Exercise 2.2 | Examining Your Attitudes and Behaviors

Instructions: In order of importance, list those attitudes and behaviors that you want to improve or change. Recognizing them will be a good start toward changing them.

Attitudes	Behaviors
1.	1.
2.	2.
3.	3.
4.	4.
5.	5.
6.	6.
7.	7.
8.	8.

Adjusting Your Attitudes

The most difficult attitudes to change are those that you have held over a long period of time. Deeply ingrained attitudes, positive or negative, create self-fulfilling prophecies. In other words, if you have a negative attitude about your ability or body, then it is likely that you will display behavior that matches your thoughts. Ultimately, all attitudes will be manifested in your behaviors. Likewise, negative attitudes about other people will lead to negative interactions with, and responses from, those people.

Attitude Adjustment Exercises

The following exercises will help you adjust your negative attitudes.

EXERCISE 2.3 USING POSITIVE LANGUAGE

Instructions: Find a quiet place. Think about the attitude you would like to adjust, and write down several statements that reflect that attitude. Then read through and consider what you wrote, ensuring that each statement accurately reflects the attitude. Next, rewrite each statement by changing the negative concepts to positive concepts. In the days that follow, make an effort to speak about yourself or others in a positive manner, and stop yourself from making negative statements. For example, you could replace "my muscular size is too small" with "my size is increasing every day as I apply the scientific methods of muscle development to my training."

EXERCISE 2.4 POSITIVE AFFIRMATIONS

Instructions: When you encounter an attitude that is difficult to change or you begin to doubt your newly adjusted attitude, stop and examine your thoughts. Restate the attitude in simple terms to help you determine if the attitude is positive or negative. If the attitude is negative, make it into a positive statement. For example, "I always lose my focus in front of spectators" could be rephrased as "I have excellent focusing skill in front of spectators." Even if they are inconsistent with your current thinking, positive statements become self-fulfilling prophecies. You can use these positive statements as daily affirmations. As you practice your positive affirmations, you will begin to replace your old self-image with the new self-image you are developing.

EXERCISE 2.5 PERSONAL INSPIRATION CARDS

Instructions: On 3 × 5 note cards, write down 10 positive statements about yourself. Each statement should be the opposite of a negative attitude you have about yourself. Carry one card with you each day, and force yourself to read it at least 10 times throughout the day. It is important that you try to believe the statement each time you read it. The more you believe each inspirational message, the more quickly you will integrate these positive attitudes in your normal pattern of thinking.

EXERCISE 2.6 REALITY CHECK

Instructions: Do you find that you train and follow your nutritional program religiously yet never seem to develop as quickly as those who seem to put in less effort? Does it seem that no matter how often you train, how much rest you get, or how low-fat your diet is, the same people always seem to achieve better results? While effective training, a healthy diet, plenty of rest, and "good" genetics certainly play a key role in body development, it is a dysfunctional attitude that holds most people back. The ideas you hold about yourself, your training partner, and even other competitors usually originate with comparison. Bodybuilders often compare their own bodies with the bodies of other bodybuilders.

Write down what you think about other bodybuilders you know. Then read and evaluate each statement in terms of how it corresponds with reality. Most likely, you have projected unrealistic qualities or attributes on other bodybuilders. For example, you may see them as better trained, more capable, or better endowed genetically. In other words, you have probably made them out to be superhuman bodybuilders who are capable of outperforming you in every area of muscular development. After careful reflection, you will begin to realize that other bodybuilders are human, each with their own strengths and weaknesses, and you will be able to restore your thinking to a realistic level.

EXERCISE 2.7 CONTROL

Instructions: If you are in a positive situation that you can control, it is important to do whatever is necessary to maintain that position. More often, however, you will find yourself uncomfortable with your surroundings and unable to control them. If you know which aspects of a situation make you uncomfortable and you understand the power you have to change them, you can deal with your negative feelings. For example, if you have the choice to use a favorite piece of exercise equipment rather than one you detest, you will likely make that choice. But when you are unable to change the situation, you must adjust your attitude to make the best of a negative situation.

You may find that you are unable to eat low-fat items as often as you like, that there are limits to how often and how long you can work out, and that your sleeping habits and patterns may not always be consistent. You have no control over a lot of these variables. The reality for most people is that they are unable to focus completely on muscular development—they have lives outside of bodybuilding. The challenge is not to give up, and not to panic at a seeming lack of control.

You must first decide which things you have control over and which things are out of your control. For example, you may not like a particular competition venue: it may be too dark, the stage may be too small, and the spectators may sit too close or too far from stage. Nevertheless, you will most likely have no control over where competitions are held and will need to overcome those problems if you are going to perform at an optimal level. You must reassure yourself and begin to transform your negative thoughts into positive ones. This also applies to training partners, gyms, food choices, and judges. No situation is going to be perfect. Approach every situation with a positive, take-charge attitude to assure yourself that even though some things are beyond your control, you can remain composed.

Personal Motivation

Motivation has received much attention in sport psychology over the years. Many sport researchers have attempted to understand the way motivation affects athletic performance, and to gain a conceptual and definitional understanding of motivation. Motivation is the product of interaction between your individual qualities and the physical and social environments in which you live and function. In other words, your motivation level is dependent on the strength of your internal motivation and the interaction that occurs between you and your physical and social environment. It is not the role of your coach, training partner, parents, or friends to motivate you; it is your job to stay motivated and committed within your environment.

Self-motivation in a winning athlete stems from two main sources: (1) self-expectant view of the world and (2) awareness that fear and desire are among the greatest motivators. Simply put, winning athletes expect that their abilities and effort will carry them to the final podium of success. They understand the more you want something, the greater sacrifice and effort you are willing to give. Desire leads to achievement, success, and satisfaction and for the bodybuilder, can lead to an enhanced body shape. Even though fear can be a great motivator, it can also be destructive and lead to poor training patterns. Keep the two main sources of self-motivation in mind and learn to focus on the rewards of success and actively tune out the fear of failure.

Everyone is motivated to some degree. The difference between a winner and a loser is that degree. A loser will say, "I have to, but I can't." A winner will say, "I want to, I can, and I will!"

Before you read on, ask yourself the following questions to begin the process of thinking about motivation and how it affects your commitment to training.

- What are my dominant fears?
- What motivating effect do these fears have in my bodybuilding?

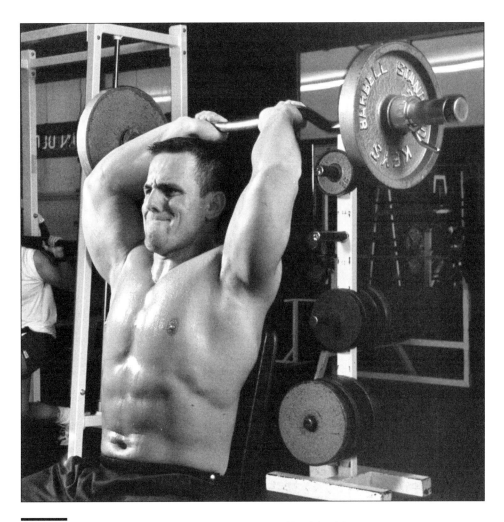

Few activities require the motivational intensity of bodybuilding.

- What are my dominant desires?
- Do I focus most of my attention and thoughts about bodybuilding on these desires?
- Do I focus on the rewards of success more than the penalties of failure?

The Motivation Continuum

The degree of one's personal motivation lies on a continuum (figure 2.1), ranging from non-motivation to intrinsic motivation. Between these two ends lies extrinsic (external) motivation, including non-self-determined and self-determined extrinsic motivation. If you understand the type of motivation you have, you can improve it and work toward a type of motivation better suited to long-term body development.

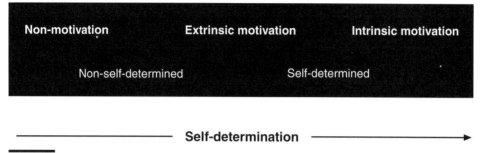

——————————————————— **Self-determination** ——————————————→

Figure 2.1   Motivation continuum.

Improving your motivation will give you a better chance of remaining committed and reaching your full potential. A brief definition of each type of motivation follows.

- Non-motivation: Bodybuilders do not know why they participate and are neither intrinsically nor extrinsically motivated.
- Non-self-determined extrinsic motivation: Bodybuilders participate for rewards and recognition, are externally regulated, and do not perceive behavior as related to their choices.
- Self-determined extrinsic motivation: Bodybuilders experience a sense of direction and purpose when training because it helps them to achieve their goals.
- Intrinsic motivation: Bodybuilders train for the inherent pleasure and satisfaction they derive from working out.

Athlete Motivation and Bodybuilders

Motivation is a psychological force that drives people to perform. You have probably seen bodybuilders who need external motivation just to get to the gym. You have also probably seen bodybuilders with a high degree of internal motivation, evidenced by their phenomenal work ethic. They have the desire to fulfill their potential and will do whatever it takes to get there.

From the mountain of research on athlete motivation, it is clear that athletes who perceive themselves as capable and in control tend to exert more effort in mastering a task, experience more positive feelings, and usually remain motivated over a longer period of time. Sure, chatting it up with someone in the gym can be fun, but does it really help you reach your goal? If you waste time or are tired, anxious, emotionally drained, or depressed in the gym, you cannot expect to get your best results. To be at your very best throughout the year, you must stay motivated. People such as your training partner or spouse will also be able to help you by creating an environment that enhances your own motivation. For example, they could give you more free time to train, drive you to the gym, and prepare meals that energize you. Intrinsically motivated bodybuilders are also good to train with, because their enthusiasm and desire rubs off on those around them.

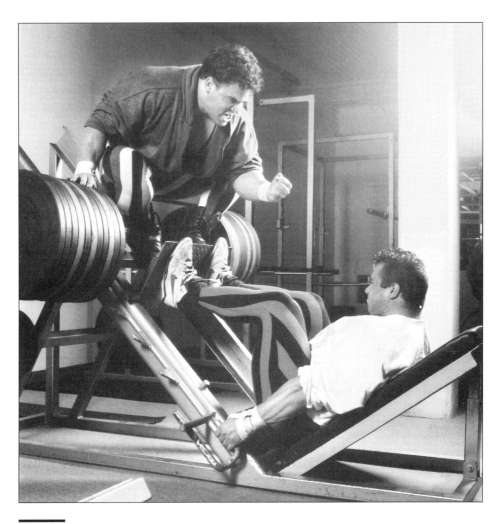

A training partner can motivate you to levels that you never dreamed of.

Interestingly enough, intrinsically motivated bodybuilders are not always the most genetically gifted. In fact, genetically gifted bodybuilders are often less intrinsically motivated, because muscular development comes easy for them. When they train, they make incredible gains most bodybuilders can only dream about. It makes you wonder, just how much could a genetically gifted bodybuilder accomplish if he or she was highly motivated and trained well?

Intrinsically motivated bodybuilders, like any intrinsically motivated athletes, are able to push past the comfort zone in training because of their internal drive to achieve their body potential. Sometimes this high level of confidence is confused with being conceited or "cocky." Provided that you are giving maximum effort and have the "right" genetics, however, there is nothing wrong with being highly confident. It should be encouraged by those around you.

Patterns of Motivation

According to Ralph Vernacchia, a leading sport psychologist, there are a number of different patterns of athletic motivation.[5] As you read through each of the different patterns of athletic motivation in exercise 2.8, decide which pattern generally reflects your motivational style and answer the questions provided with that pattern.

Exercise 2.8 | Patterns of Motivation

MOTIVATION PATTERN #1: LEARNED HELPLESSNESS

These bodybuilders believe that no matter how hard they try, the outcome is beyond their control. They lack effort and discipline in both training and lifestyle practices. They attribute success or failure to external factors beyond their control, such as the genetic quality of other bodybuilders or luck. Acquired through experience and faulty guidance, learned helplessness is usually found in novice bodybuilders, but it can also be present in those who have been lifting for years. Bodybuilders with this type of motivation must understand that they do have control over many aspects of their body development and that even small achievements must be considered successes.

1. How do you define *success* in terms of personal improvement of your own body?

   _____

   _____

2. List two or three past successes, and include the steps that led to success.

   _____

   _____

3. List two or three short-term goals for bodybuilding, and identify small successes you have enjoyed, such as adding weight to your bench press or making every workout in the past month.

   _____

   _____

MOTIVATION PATTERN #2: FEAR OF FAILURE

These bodybuilders are primarily motivated by a fear of failure, which not only is a major source of stress but takes the enjoyment out of the sport, creating a tentative and tenuous training style. Fear of failure results when positive feedback is conditional and the use of rewards is inappropriate. These bodybuilders usually measure their self-worth in terms of "winning" or "losing," both external comparisons, but they must understand that every athlete fails to reach some goals. Learning from failure is what counts.

1. Identify two or three talents outside of bodybuilding.

   _____

   _____

2. List the two or three most developed features of your body. How do these features compare to those of other bodybuilders?

   _____

   _____

3. List any thoughts you have about the formula of success: Success = effort $\times$ preparation $\times$ will $\times$ genetic makeup.

   _____

   _____

MOTIVATION PATTERN #3: FEAR OF SUCCESS

Like fear of failure, fear of success can be a major source of stress for any athlete. These bodybuilders are preoccupied with the negative aspects of being successful bodybuilders. For example, they experience too much pressure from competitors; they get messages from trainers and others that they need to improve; they are the object of jealousy; and they have the responsibility of being role models. In other words, fear of success is the over riding concern that success may lead to external stressors that are too difficult to manage. Low self-worth can also contribute to fear of success. For these bodybuilders, it is important to remember that they are what they think. Negative beliefs about your ability to succeed will most likely be realized. Learn to pursue your own goals, and put the expectations of others into perspective.

1. What will it take to be the one of the best bodybuilders in your gym, in your city, in your region, or in your country?

   _____

   _____

(continued)

2. What will it take to stay in peak physical condition?

_____

_____

3. If you were highly successful, what attitudes would you expect to see from other gym members, your training partner, other competitors, and other significant people in your life? How would you respond to those attitudes?

_____

_____

MOTIVATION PATTERN #4: PERFECTIONISM

These bodybuilders expect consistently superior performance, which is nearly impossible for even the best bodybuilders. Such expectations mean little, if any, success and lead to dissatisfaction in training. Perfectionistic bodybuilders believe that every workout should be great and that they should never cheat on their diets. They even blame themselves for hitting strength and size plateaus.

Virtually no one could live up to those expectations. These bodybuilders need to develop an appreciation for rest and relaxation, and understand that all athletes make mistakes. By redefining failure and avoiding negative language, even perfectionistic bodybuilders can learn to enjoy the success that comes from hard work.

1. Determine an acceptable number of poor workouts or cheats on your diet in a month. Is this number reasonable?

_____

_____

2. Talk to your personal trainer or training partner and find out how many failures he or she thinks is reasonable for a bodybuilder at your level. Write that number here.

_____

_____

3. Talk to other bodybuilders and find out how much time they spend each week in training and preparation of nutritious meals. Is your time commitment in line with theirs?

_____

_____

MOTIVATION PATTERN #5: UNDERACHIEVEMENT

These bodybuilders have little appreciation for the hard work and self-discipline required in successful bodybuilding. Although many are genetically gifted, underachievers never really develop an understanding of their true potential. They often enjoy early success in bodybuilding, but as they begin to compete at higher levels, their lack of training soon catches up to them. Genetically inferior bodybuilders, who have trained hard for longer periods of time, begin to pass them by. Bodybuilders who lean toward underachievement must commit to changing their attitudes and then take the necessary steps to ensure success, such as greater training intensity, adequate sleep, healthy eating, and consultation with personal trainers and support people.

1. What has allowed you to create the body you now have?

_____

_____

2. What can you do to ensure that you will be able to develop to your potential?

_____

_____

3. Based on your body and capacity to gain muscular size and definition, set some goals for yourself. Do not compare what you achieve with what others achieve, because you are probably capable of accomplishing much more than that.

_____

_____

(continued)

MOTIVATION PATTERN #6: LEARNED EFFECTIVENESS

These bodybuilders believe they are successful because they are determined and in control. They have the will and the commitment to pursue clearly defined goals, and they attribute success or failure to such factors as effort, genetics, and discipline. These bodybuilders have no motivational problems and are encouraged to continue in this pattern.

1. How were you able to develop this motivational pattern?

   _____

   _____

2. Without causing stress or tension, in what ways could you encourage others in your gym to develop this type of motivational pattern?

   _____

   _____

3. Do you have any weaknesses that you would like to work on over the next few months?

   _____

   _____

Tips for Improving Motivation

The following are some tips for improving your motivation:

- Replace the word *can't* with *can* in your daily vocabulary. *Can* applies to 90 percent of the challenges that you face, both in life and in bodybuilding.
- Replace the word *try* with *will* in your daily vocabulary. When you *try* something, you have a built-in excuse for failure.
- Create a self-fulfilling prophecy. Focus your attention and energy on achieving the bodybuilding goals you have established. Forget about the consequences of failure. Remember, you usually get what you think most about.
- List five of your most important desires in bodybuilding. Next to each one, list the benefit or payoff you will get when you achieve it. Look at

this list before you go to bed each night and when you get up each morning.

- Find an expert. If there is something you want to do or experience as a bodybuilder but are afraid to try, find someone who is currently doing what you want to do and talk to him or her. Perhaps you want to change your workouts or start using a vitamin supplement. Perhaps you are thinking about entering your first competition, turning professional, or becoming a personal trainer. Get the facts. Make a project of learning everything you can from bodybuilders you identify as winners.

- Develop a new vocabulary for talking about yourself. For every one of your goals, make it a habit to repeat again and again, "I want to—I can. I want to—I can!"

- Motivate others. When motivating training partners, paint the picture of what achievement looks and feels like, and demonstrate your confidence and belief in their ability to accomplish their goals. Rather than say, "It is almost impossible for you to make those muscular gains," motivate them: "I have noticed your commitment to your diet. Keep up the hard work. It is really beginning to pay off."

- Deal with your fear. It is normal to worry, certainly, but doing so can negatively affect your motivation for bodybuilding. Besides, we most often worry about things that will never happen. Communication and understanding can go a long way in transforming worry into positive, action-directed thinking. Start by dealing with the issues underlying your fears. For example, if you are worried what your spouse will think of your commitment to bodybuilding, it would be best to sit down and talk with him or her about it.

- Stay positive. When your training partner tells you his or her problems, respond with solution-orientated feedback. When you are having problems, focus on finding the answer.

- Stay focused. When you set new goals or start a bodybuilding project, concentrate all of your energy and intensity, without distraction, on the successful completion of that goal or project.

Adapted from Waitley 1987.[6]

Emotional Intelligence

Why is it that some bodybuilders always seem to win and others always seem to lose? Why is it that some people never seem to miss a workout and are always able to stick to a healthy, muscle-building nutrition program? People who rise to the top of their fields—whether psychology, law, medicine, engineering, or coaching—are proficient at more than their occupation.

They are usually affable, resilient, and optimistic. Put another way, it takes more than a high IQ to be successful. It also takes "emotional intelligence" (EQ), including the ability to let go of negative feelings and instead focus on the positive.

Think back to high school, when you knew which kids would become the most successful adults. You probably looked to the students with the highest intellectual credentials: the ones with the best grades, those heading to college or university, or those with the highest IQs. Where are those students now? Sure, some of them may have become successful in business, sport, and relationships, but did all of them achieve such success? And what about the students without high intellectual credentials? Believe it or not, IQ accounts for a mere 20 percent in determining success, leaving a whopping 80 percent to other factors. In other words, when it comes to life's most challenging moments, you need other types of resourcefulness. EQ gives you a competitive edge.

After reading Daniel Goleman's book *Emotional Intelligence: Why It Can Matter More than IQ*,[7] I started thinking, "If emotional intelligence seems to give people an edge in the academic and business arenas, what about sport? Would bodybuilders with a high EQ be more successful than those without?" According to Dr. Steven Stein, clinical psychologist, president of Multi-Health Systems (MHS), and publisher of the first scientific measure of EQ, "Emotional intelligence is an important factor for winning athletes. What separates star-performing athletes from the rest is their ability to be in touch with their emotions and to channel them as needed. This means having good impulse control and an optimistic outlook on life."

According to the book *Emotional Development and Emotional Intelligence*,[8] emotional intelligence involves "the ability to monitor one's own and others emotions, discriminate among them, and . . . use that information to guide one's thinking and actions." These are the key components in successful bodybuilding. Because bodybuilding is a highly emotional sport, participants must control their emotions and use them to assist in their training.

Bodybuilding and EQ

EQ is a psychological construct consisting of 15 different factors, many of which are not directly related to bodybuilding. Five of those factors, however, are crucial in developing a fit, muscular body in a short amount of time. Three of these factors have already been discussed, namely, self-awareness, motivation, and self-confidence. The two remaining factors are outlined here.

- Intentionality: The desire and capacity to make an impact, and to act with persistence. If you desire to make an impact on the beach, in the gym, or at a bodybuilding competition, you will need to have an intentional focus of determination and persistence. Bodybuilders with high EQ have the ability to train with intention to a stronger degree than those with low EQ.

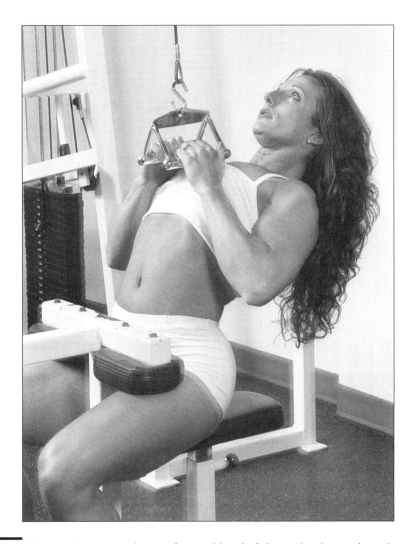

Intentionality requires you to have a focused level of determination and persistence.

- Self-control: The ability to temper and control one's actions appropriately. You will need to get plenty of rest, eat muscle-building foods, and train with great intensity if you are going to create the body you want. Managing your emotions and self-discipline is a must to be a successful bodybuilder.

Now I will let you in on a little secret: EQ is not something you have to be born with. According to Dr. Stein, "Emotional skills can be trained and improved—think of it as improving the muscle in your mind. In this case it means using your lower brain to produce high performance."

Improving Your EQ

If you want to improve your EQ for bodybuilding then I suggest that you focus on the four areas of motivation, confidence, intentionality, and self-awareness. This section provides tips and advice on how to make deliberate efforts for change. For information on how to improve self-awareness and personal motivation, see exercises 1.2, 1.3 and 2.8.

Confidence.   Step back and reevaluate each small step you have taken in training. For example, if you think you will never be able to bench press 300 pounds, look at the steps you have outlined to get there, such as increasing each set by 10 pounds at a time. Increasing by smaller increments, say, only 5 pounds each set, might yield greater success. The smaller the steps, the greater your success, and the more confident you will be.

Look around and see what others are doing. See how well you are doing when compared to most people. If your progress is behind that of other bodybuilders then you will know what you must do. If you are further ahead then you can use that to build your confidence.

Intentionality.   What is your dream goal? What do you want to accomplish in the next five years? Affirm these goals, no matter what people say about them. All goals will eventually be subject to a reality check but allow yourself to "dream" when you set dream goals. I tell my students that they can accomplish whatever they want in life if they just put their hearts and minds to it. Society needs brain surgeons and rocket scientists and there is no reason why most people couldn't have those aspirations. There are professional bodybuilders capable of making a good living, even winning the Mr. Olympic contest, why not you?

Set challenges for yourself—a great lift, larger biceps, or completing the toughest treadmill level. Then go for it and allow nothing to get in the way of meeting that challenge. Do not let depression, worry, and anger paralyze the joy of being super-fit.

Self-Control.   Learn to delay gratification. Consider the famous marshmallow test: A researcher placed a marshmallow in front of four-year-old children and said, "You can have this marshmallow now, if you want, but if you wait until I run an errand, you can have two." A third of the kids ate the marshmallow, a third waited for a while but then ate the marshmallow, and the other third waited until the researcher came back. When subjects were contacted 14 years later, the early "grabbers" were still impulsive and very quick to anger, while the "waiters" were popular and emotionally balanced. The late "grabbers" were more emotionally balanced than the early "grabbers" but not nearly as controlled as the "waiters." Amazingly enough, the "waiters" tended to score higher on their SAT scores.

Learn to control yourself when it comes to eating unhealthy foods, consistently staying up late, or missing essential workouts. If you are easily angered or frustrated, stop what you are doing and take a deep breath. Count slowly to 10, and then resume your activity. This will allow you time to relax and think of an appropriate action before making a fool of yourself.

CHAPTER 3

Grasping the Essential Mind-Body Connection

It only takes a cursory glance at the history of philosophy to understand the difficulty presented by the interdependence of the mind and body. Since the writings of Descartes more than three centuries ago, the philosophical world has been in turmoil over the issue of the mind-body connection. Descartes concluded that man is made up of two distinct substances: body and mind. The body was viewed as an unthinking, material substance that conformed to the mechanical laws of nature. The mind was a thinking, immaterial substance that was not susceptible to the mechanical laws of nature. Each was considered a distinct, independent entity.

This approach is smattered with difficulties. Of course the mind and body are interrelated. Cognitive and emotional qualities cannot exist without a corresponding physical sensation, and vice versa. For example, while it may be possible to distinguish between the emotional qualities and physical sensations of pain, they are related and they work together. The same is true for other human sensations, such as thirst, hunger, and sex.

Given this interrelation, can you imagine the mind not being involved in bodybuilding, never experiencing the joy of a completed set, the happiness of placing in a bodybuilding contest, or even the disappointment of a missed lift or the frustration of an injury? Every bodybuilder knows that such mental states as excitement and elation produce noticeable changes in the cardiovascular and respiratory systems, the muscular frame, and in the degree of intensity during a set or workout. Clearly, a human being, a unity of physical, biological, and psychological relationships, only makes sense when it is considered as a whole.

Most bodybuilders separate the mind and body when they engage in training, adopting the "mind over matter" philosophy and pushing through with their plans to "correct" or alter the body. While it is indeed possible for the mind to control the body, this is not the optimal view of the mind-body relationship. Rather, the mind and body working together create a total immersion in the workout, fostering an environment in which bodybuilders can experience their power, become aware of their capabilities and limitations, and affirm their dynamic mind-body connection. Then and only then will bodybuilders get the most out of their workouts.

Most people approach bodybuilding as a way to improve the fitness and look of the body, giving little attention to the brain. But, as already discussed, mental power is more important for effective training than mere genetics and body function. While body-orientated training programs are usually well developed, there is definitely room for improvement where mental training is concerned. Indeed, the deciding factor in a well-organized and effective training program is often mental.

Mind–Body Communication

Ultimately, it is the quality of the mind-body relationship and the degree to which you maintain harmony and cooperation between them that will set you apart from others. Bodybuilders who learn to listen to their bodies tap into their full potential for body development and shaping. Unfortunately, bodybuilders tend not to be good listeners. Statements such as "I am just going to learn to ignore my thoughts completely," or even "I am not going to allow myself to feel pain," indicate a problematic future, if not imminent training plateaus. The reality is, neither of these strategies is effective. If you ignore your thoughts, they will find a way of intruding, distorting, or distracting you from the task at hand. On the other hand, shutting out all physical signals can lead to serious physical injury and mental relapse.

Every bodybuilder is familiar with mental excuses for not working out: "I am tired, so I will just go home," "I worked hard last time, so I will just go easy today," "I will never get any bigger, so what's the use," and so on. These thoughts, expressed in gyms across the world, are nothing but a cancer to goal accomplishment. The correct approach is to develop a balance between mind and body in such a way that both have equal influence toward success.

Establishing that connection first involves improving the communication between body and mind. While this certainly includes using the mind to help direct and motivate the body, it is crucial that the needs of the body be considered and responded to. In their book *Sporting Body Sporting Mind,* John Syer and Christopher Connolly write, "effective communication is a two-way process: if you are to communicate properly with your body, you must

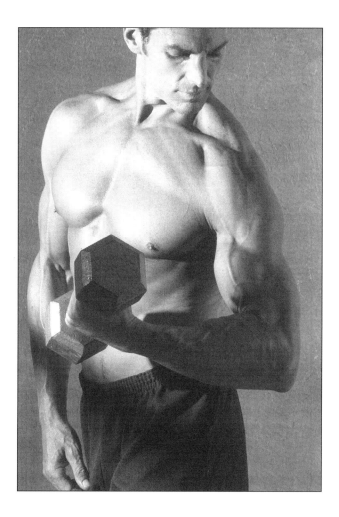

A sophisticated relationship exists between your mind and body.

understand what your body is saying to you. . . . To educate your body, you must know how it functions and learn its language." They go on to explain that educating your body involves four key processes: learning, training, maintenance, and change.[1]

Learning

From the day that you are born, you continually improve your physical performance. Walking evolves into running, which eventually evolves into specific running skills in sport. Likewise, other skills, such as throwing a ball, reading, and brushing your teeth, continue to improve throughout childhood and adolescence. These skills involve a learning process. Physical skills require learning to use your body and manipulate your environment, and mental skills require learning to use your mind.

It has been said that bodybuilding is for those lacking the mental fortitude to engage in any other sport. Nothing could be farther from the truth. To develop the desired look, bodybuilders must learn how to use their bodies and minds effectively. Bodybuilding is a complex activity that encompasses many different techniques and skills. How do you pick out a novice at the gym? Not just by the black socks in white runners. Beginners stick out by their obvious lack of direction and incorrect lifting techniques. They simply look out of place. They have not yet learned the unique culture of the gym and how lifting exercises are to be performed.

Training

An incredibly sophisticated, yet remarkably simple relationship exists between the nervous and muscular system and the rest of the body. Each physical move sends thousands of signals per second to the brain, which in turn unifies them into a cohesive whole. The brain then makes the appropriate decisions and sends specific messages back through the nervous system to individual muscle fibers, glands, and organs. The brain and the individual muscle fibers continue this pattern of reciprocal communication for the duration of the contraction. For repeated muscle contractions, this series of communications is repeated for seconds, minutes, or hours, depending on the duration of the exercise. Some contractions are weak and finely controlled (such as handwriting), while others are generally controlled and forceful (such as lifting weights).

During the training process, a number of neuromuscular adaptations must occur to accommodate increases in strength, power, and muscle mass. While new information about the relationship between the nervous system and the muscular system is always being discovered, it is clear that different training protocols have different effects on that relationship. Current research seems to indicate that long time athletes engaged in high-intensity, low-volume powerlifting programs may already have reached a high percentage of adaptational capacity in their muscle fibers. This means that the low exercise volume is not enough to stimulate further enlargement of the muscles. So, even though strength is developed in high-intensity, low-volume programs, they are simply not appropriate to stimulate muscle hypertrophy (increased muscle size). Conversely, high-volume, moderate-intensity training programs, like bodybuilding, develop muscle mass, which enhances the body's natural anabolic hormonal responses to training. Muscle hypertrophy, rather than strength, is emphasized, and neural factors play a smaller role in the adaptation.[2]

Maintenance and Change

Human beings are creatures of habit. Look around the gym, and it becomes evident that most people follow the same program week after week—always warming up on the same exercise bike and using the same piece of equipment each session. Why? People prefer familiar surroundings. Indeed, even the thought of making a change creates stress in many people. The same is true of bodybuilders, and not just beginners. Nevertheless, to improve your physique, you must be able to discriminate between the part of your lifting technique that is helpful and the part that is not.

Keeping the habits that work and changing those that do not work is called "maintenance." At the outset, it would seem that there is nothing wrong with that. For the bodybuilder, however, there is really no such thing as maintenance. In an adult, muscles are either increasing in size and strength or doing just the opposite. That is, muscles are either in a state of hypertrophy or in a state of atrophy. They cannot do both.

Because bodybuilding is largely about change, nothing produces failure like success. Success can cause bodybuilders to blindly stick with their exercise routines, even if those routines are no longer beneficial. Just because the cable curl helped to shape your biceps in the past, there is no guarantee that progress will continue forever. Your body will go through many different changes as it adapts to your training program. It will grow and develop, but it will also reach plateaus. Exercises that worked in the past may not be as effective now.

Rather than maintain the same workout schedule and become discouraged by training plateaus, learn to make appropriate changes—use different exercises, try different numbers of sets and reps, train less or more often, combine intense workouts with easier workouts, and use a variety of workout programs such as Olympic lifting, circuit training, and plyometrics. This is what periodization is all about: changing your training program so that your body continues to develop and grow.

Establishing Mind-Body Communication

Bodybuilding is unique in the sports world. Bodybuilders are probably more knowledgeable about their bodies, nutrition, and physiology, and they are more likely to be committed to good lifestyle patterns than are other athletes. They learn the most effective ways to train their bodies to ensure maximum growth and symmetry. Cultivating good lifting habits is only part of the program, however. Bodybuilders must invest in the process of self-discovery by creating innovative lifting techniques and sets.

Successful bodybuilders understand the powerful mind-body communication that occurs during a typical workout, set, or repetition. They realize that bodybuilding is great not only for physical fitness but also for recharging mentally and emotionally. Adding a mind-body component to a workout can provide greater intensity, relaxation, and stress management for a bodybuilder. It can also offer the opportunity for positive visualization, which can significantly improve goal attainment in health, fitness, and body image. The following tips will help you turn a routine workout into an invigorating, enlightening experience.

- Begin by noticing your breathing. Feel your rib cage expand and contract with each breath. Take a few deep breaths, and then begin to focus on exhaling and inhaling deeply with each contraction.

- Feel your muscles contract and relax with each rep. Notice the size expansion as blood begins to flow to each working muscle. Stay with the rhythm of the set, and imagine yourself pumping with confidence through life.

- Bring your awareness to other parts of your body—legs, waist, hips, and face. Feel how they adjust to the exercise and how they stabilize your movement. Know that your entire body is working together to make you stronger and more alive. Imagine that you are moving through your life with complete body synchronicity.

- Focus on the center of your body, imagining that all your strength originates there. Visualize the muscle-building energy flowing from your center to your working muscles. Imagine that puppet strings are attached to your limbs as you visualize a puppeteer helping you to lift the weight.

- As you finish your set, expand your awareness to include everything around you. Notice every piece of equipment, person, smell, and fluctuation in temperature. See yourself in the gym as the center of attraction.

- Empower yourself with positive affirmations. Feel your power, strength, and muscles. You are in peak condition. Affirm your body with silent statements, such as "I love my strong, ripped physique," or "I feel and look awesome." See yourself as the bodybuilder you want to be, and believe that you will get there.

Mind–Body Interplay During Workouts

It is now obvious that your body goes through many physiological and psychological changes during exercise. What may not be so obvious is that while you are training, there is a continuous, almost subconscious interplay between your mind and body. This interplay, positive or negative, plays a significant role in determining the ultimate success of your workouts. Understanding this interplay, including how to adjust your thinking so that it does not negatively affect your workouts, is essential for every body-builder. Tables 3.1, 3.2, and 3.3 describe mind-body interplay during three exercises: the bench press, barbell curl, and squat. These examples do not include every conceivable mind-body interaction, of course, but they should give you a good idea of the complexity of the interplay.

Mind and Body Connection: Bill Luke

Bill Luke, PhD, CSCS, is an avid weight trainer, hockey coach, fitness enthusiast, and professor at Trinity Western University in Langley, British Columbia, Canada. He has worked with many individuals and teams in strength and conditioning development. Bill is the owner of and consultant with Performance Master Consultants, a Langley-based company that trains strength and conditioning professionals. His time as an elite hockey coach and 15 years as a professor have given him a unique awareness of the critical relationship between physical performance and mental strength. Bill shares his insights about the mind-body connection below:

As a sport physiologist and conditioning coach, I have worked with many competitive athletes and fitness enthusiasts in developing resistance-training and total-body-conditioning programs. Well-designed and well-implemented resistance training (i.e., bodybuilding) plays a major role in the physical and psychological health of individuals. Indeed, there is a clear and identifiable relationship between feeling good, looking good, and having a positive self-image and self-esteem. Strong self-confidence and positive self-esteem create a psychological well-being that results in the ability to face new challenges in competition, career, relationships, and day-to-day life.

The results of training—including increased muscle strength and power; enhanced sport performance; improved physical appearance and stress management; and increased positive hormonal response—all produce self-confidence and a positive outlook on life. Research also indicates that physical self-confidence contributes significantly to positive social interaction and comfort.

Have you ever heard the saying "the rich get richer and the poor get poorer?" Well the same thing happens with the mind-body relationship. If you have ever felt healthy, strong, and satisfied with what you see in the mirror, I am sure there was a corresponding sense of physical and psychological competence, along with a greater willingness to engage in and adhere to a program of physical activity. In other words, the better you feel about yourself, the more likely it is that you will want to keep improving your physique, whether it be through weight training, bodybuilding, cardio-vascular training, or any other recreational or competitive pursuit.

The psychological benefits that result from weight lifting and bodybuilding cannot be ignored. Regardless of one's motivation for beginning a weight-training or bodybuilding program, the mind and body become intimately linked during training, and this soon carries over to time spent away from the gym. The best part is, these benefits are available to anyone who engages in strength training. What more could anyone ask for?

Table 3.1 Mind-Body Interplay During the Bench Press

Action	Mind response	Body response
You lie down on the bench and get ready to grip the bar.	• "I see myself as being strong and capable of pushing through the expected pain." • "I know I am capable of lifting this weight."	• Anticipation increases heart and breathing rates. • Blood pressure rises, and adrenal glands increase the secretion of adrenaline.
You adjust your grip to get just the right feel.	• "The bar must feel right in my hands." • "I must be ready to lift, and adjusting my grip gives me a few seconds to narrow my focus."	• Skin sensors alert the brain that the bar needs to be re-gripped for maximum comfort. • Adrenaline levels cause the heart to beat faster and contract more forcefully.
As you lift the bar off the rack, the weight presses heavily against your palms.	• "I am ready; now is the time to perform and be ready." • "The weight does feel heavy in my hands, but it will feel better after the first rep." • "I am going to take a few deep breaths, concentrate, and get ready to powerfully execute this set."	• Adrenaline is at peak level. • Maximum pressure is felt against the palms, telling the brain that the weight is heavy. • Stimulation of the motor nerves results in propagation of action potentials to the muscle fibers of the chest muscles.
You lower the bar toward your chest and press up again.	• "I must move the bar in a smooth and controlled manner." • "I will maintain my focus by directing my eyes toward the bar and taking control of the bar." • "I can feel my chest muscles stretch as the bar approaches my chest, and I feel my arms power through as I push the bar away."	• The heart begins to pump more blood to the chest muscles. • The chest muscles stretch to prepare for the powerful contraction during the lifting phase.

Action	Mind response	Body response
Each succeeding repetition feels heavier and heavier.	• "I am really starting to feel tired, and each rep is getting more difficult." • "Push through, keep strong, maintain focus. This is difficult, but I can make it."	• The heart is pumping maximum volumes of blood to the working muscles, aided by the dilated coronary arteries. • The motor unit (muscle fiber and Aα motor nerve) contracts with increasing force. • Fast-twitch glycolic muscle fibers begin to tire from lactate production.
Your breathing is forced and rhythmically timed with each rep.	• "My breathing keeps my mind on the task." • "Exhaling during the lifting phase and inhaling during the recovery phase help me lift with greater efficiency."	• Blood lactate begins to accumulate and acidosis begins to develop, causing fatigue.
The bar moves slowly on the last rep as the weight is pressing against you.	• "Keep pressing. Do not give up, no matter how hard it seems." • "There is no danger, because my training partner is there for me." • "It is the most intense repetitions that force the muscle to grow."	• Blood lactate reaches maximum level and the fast-twitch glycolic muscle fibers reach maximum fatigue. • The motor unit (muscle fiber and Aα motor nerve) contracts with maximum force. • Fast-twitch glycolic muscle fibers reach maximum fatigue from lactate production. • Creatine phospate (CrP) is almost completely depleted.

(continued)

Table 3.2 *(continued)*

Action	Mind response	Body response
You place the bar back onto the rack, take a deep breath, and let your arms fall down to your sides.	• "It feels so good to have completed that set." • "The blood is really rushing to my chest, and I can really feel the pump." • "I am so glad that I completed that set with focused intensity. Now my chest can really grow."	• Muscles begin the recovery process while maintaining small amounts of motor unit contraction to maintain skeletal muscle tone. • The blood begins the process of flushing out the lactate buildup in the muscles. • CrP stores recover, and ATP regeneration occurs in the working muscles.

Table 3.2 Mind–Body Interplay During the Barbell Curl

Action	Mind response	Body response
You look into the mirror with the bar at your feet.	• "I see myself as being strong and capable of pushing through the expected pain." • "I know I am capable of curling this weight."	• Anticipation increases heart and breathing rates. • Blood pressure rises, and adrenal glands increase the secretion of adrenaline.
You pick up the bar and adjust your grip as necessary.	• "The bar must feel right in my hands." • "I must be ready to lift, and adjusting my grip gives me a few seconds to narrow my focus." • "I am ready to work hard and really pump up my biceps."	• Skin sensors alert the brain that the bar needs to be re-gripped for maximum comfort. • Adrenaline levels cause the heart to beat faster and contract more forcefully. • Neural patterns begin to develop in the motor cortex to eventually cause muscle contraction. • Adrenaline is at peak level. • The biceps prepare for the first contraction.

Action	Mind response	Body response
The first repetition is initiated and executed.	• "It seems light now, but I know that it will get heavier as I do more repetitions." • "I must keep my breathing relaxed and focused." • "I must move the bar in a smooth and controlled manner." • "I will maintain my focus by directing my eyes toward the mirror and watching my form."	• Stimulation of the motor nerves results in propagation of action potentials to the muscle fibers of the chest muscles. • The heart begins to pump more blood to the chest muscles.
Each succeeding repetition feels heavier and heavier.	• "I am really starting to feel tired, and each rep is getting more difficult." • "Push through, keep strong, maintain focus. This is difficult, but I can make it." • "I do not want to cheat. I must keep focused and force my biceps to do the work."	• The heart is pumping maximum volumes of blood to the working muscles, aided by the dilated coronary arteries. • The motor unit (muscle fiber and $A\alpha$ motor nerve) contracts with increasing force. • Fast-twitch glycolic muscle fibers begin to tire from lactate production. • Amino acid release from the working muscles is increased.
Your breathing is forced and rhythmically timed with each rep.	• "My breathing keeps my mind on the task." • "Exhaling during the lifting phase and inhaling during the recovery phase help me lift with greater efficiency."	• Blood lactate begins to accumulate and acidosis begins to develop, causing fatigue. • Mitochondrial respiration increases very quickly, affecting ATP levels.

(continued)

Table 3.2 *(continued)*

Action	Mind response	Body response
The bar feels immovable as you try to complete the final repetition.	• "Keep going. I have to keep going, even though it seems like I am not even moving the weight." • "My biceps feel like they are about to explode and rip through my skin." • "Even though I am in pain, I know that it is the most intense repetitions that force the muscle to grow."	• Blood lactate reaches maximum level and the fast-twitch glycolic muscle fibers reach maximum fatigue. • Blood glucose concentration, muscle blood flow, and muscle and blood lactate levels are all near maximum, and several substrates of glycolosis have accumulated in the muscles. • Creatine phospate (CrP) is almost completely depleted. • Micro-tears begin to appear in the working muscles.
You place the bar back on the floor and sit down in an exhausted state.	• "It feels so good to have completed that set." • "Blood is filling my biceps and my skin is so tight." • "I am so glad that I completed that set with focused intensity. Now my biceps will be able to grow."	• Excess postexercise oxygen consumption (EPOC) is highly elevated. • Muscle and blood lactate concentrations begin the process of returning to normal. • Heart and breathing rates slow down. • CrP stores recover, and ATP regeneration occurs in the working muscles.

Table 3.3	Mind–Body Interplay During the Squat	
Action	**Mind response**	**Body response**
You look into the mirror with the bar sitting on the squat rack.	• "I have very strong legs, and this weight is not going to stop me from reaching my goals." • "I know that I can push this weight up, even though it will feel heavy on my back."	• Anticipation increases heart and breathing rates. • Blood pressure rises, and adrenal glands increase the secretion of adrenaline. • Your eyes focus on the mirror and your body in the same way that your mind is focused.
You get under bar and feel the pressure of the bar against your back.	• "The bar must sit just right on my back, and my grip must feel balanced." • "I will shuffle my feet as I narrow my focus to the task at hand." • "I am ready to drive hard against this weight."	• Skin sensors alert the brain that the bar is sitting correctly on your back for maximum comfort. • Adrenaline levels cause the heart to beat faster and contract more forcefully. • Neural patterns begin to develop in the motor cortex to eventually cause muscle contraction. • Adrenaline is at peak level. • The quadriceps prepare for the first contraction.
You stand up with the weight pressing against your back and you look in the mirror.	• "This is my last chance to focus." • "I feel strong and powerful, and I am ready to execute the first rep." • "I am going to take a few deep breaths, concentrate, and get ready to powerfully execute this set."	• Adrenaline is at peak level. • Maximum pressure is felt against the back, and the legs are wobbling as the stabilizer muscles kick into high gear.

(continued)

Table 3.3 *(continued)*

Action	Mind response	Body response
The first repetition is initiated and executed.	• "It seems light now, but I know that it will get heavier as I do more repetitions." • "I must keep my breathing relaxed and focused." • "I must keep my chin up, look into the mirror, and move in a smooth, controlled manner."	• Stimulation of the motor nerves results in propagation of action potentials to the muscles fibers of the quadriceps muscles. • The heart begins to pump more blood to the working muscles as they prepare for more intense work.
Each succeeding repetition feels heavier and heavier.	• "I can really feel the burning in my legs, but I know that I can handle it." • "Push through, keep strong, maintain focus. This is difficult, but I can make it." • "I must make sure that I execute the full range of motion. If I cheat now, I will only be disappointed."	• The heart is pumping maximum volumes of blood to the working muscles, aided by the dilated coronary arteries. • The motor unit (muscle fiber and Aα motor nerve) contracts with increasing force. • Fast-twitch glycolic muscle fibers begin to tire from lactate production. • Amino acid release from the working muscles is increased.
Your breathing is forced and rhythmically timed with each rep.	• "My breathing keeps my mind on the task." • "Exhaling during the lifting phase and inhaling during the recovery phase help me lift with greater efficiency."	• Blood lactate begins to accumulate and acidosis begins to develop, causing fatigue. • Mitochondrial respiration increases very quickly, affecting ATP levels.

Action	Mind response	Body response
The bar feels immovable as you try to complete the final repetition.	• "Keep going. I have to keep going, even though it seems like I am not even moving the weight." • "My quadriceps are really burning, and it feels like the weight is pushing me into the ground. I must continue to drive hard against the weight to be succesful." • "Even though I am in pain, I know that it is the most intense repetitions that force the muscle to grow."	• Blood lactate reaches maximum level and the fast-twitch glycolic muscle fibers reach maximum fatigue. • Blood glucose concentration, muscle blood flow, and muscle and blood lactate levels are all near maximum, and several substrates of glycolosis have accumulated in the muscles. • Creatine phospate (CrP) is almost completely depleted. • Micro-tears begin to appear in the working muscles.
You place the bar back on the rack and sit down. Your legs are exhausted.	• "It feels so good to have completed that set." • "My legs feel like jelly." • "I am so glad that I completed that set with focused intensity. Now my quadriceps will be able to grow."	• Excess postexercise oxygen consumption (EPOC) is highly elevated. • Muscle and blood lactate concentrations begin the process of returning to normal. • Heart and breathing rates slow down. • CrP stores recover, and ATP regeneration occurs in the working muscles.

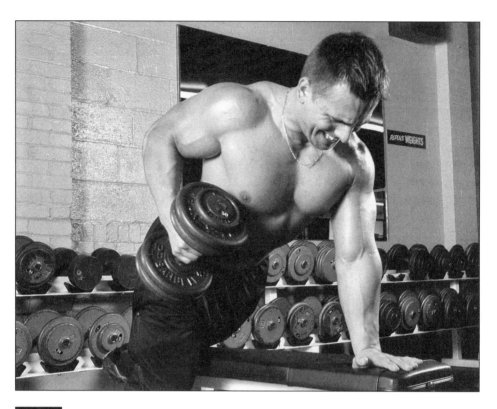

Repetions spark the subconscious interplay between your mind and your body.

Hormonal and Metabolic Response to Pumping Iron

During exercise, the body must respond rapidly to the increased demands being placed on it. The muscles have an increased need for energy, blood flow, and ventilation to circulate oxygen and remove wastes; heat must be redistributed to the periphery of the body; and fluids must be preserved to maintain appropriate cardiovascular function. These adaptations to exercise, among others, are regulated by the autonomic nervous system and hormonal glands. It is the job of the hormones to maintain normal conditions when the body is under stress, including increased glucose absorption into muscle cells, water re-absorption from kidney ducts, and muscle contraction.

During resistance training, muscles must synthesize new proteins and incorporate those proteins into an existing or newly created sarcomere. Hormones are ultimately responsible for an increase in the amount of a muscle's contractile proteins, actin and myson, which is critical for significant muscle adaptation. The stimulation of protein synthesis, the first step in muscle growth, is promoted and enhanced through heavy resistance training, allowing the muscle to become stronger and bigger. The change in muscle fiber involves a corresponding change in protein metabolism. The more muscle fibers involved in a particular exercise, the greater the degree of change within the whole muscle. This relationship between hormones and muscle fibers, and the subsequent changes in functional capability of the muscle cells, provides the basis for the adaptive influence of hormones.[3]

Understanding the natural anabolic activity that takes place in the bodybuilder's body is fundamental to successful recovery, adaptation, program design, training progression, and ultimately to body development. Although resistance training is the only form of exercise that can have a direct impact on the size and strength of a muscle group, not all resistance exercise has the same effect. Significant differences can exist among different resistance training programs in their effectiveness to increase muscle and connective tissue size and in their ability to stimulate hormonal concentrations.

Responsible for regulating many different physiological systems, hormones are chemical messengers that are synthesized by, stored in, and released by endocrine glands and other cells. Hormones typically play multiple roles, also acting as a regulatory agent for metabolic function through the control of energy substrates and nutrition absorption in cells. Hormones of interest to the bodybuilder can generally be classified in two categories: anabolic hormones and catabolic hormones. Anabolic hormones are those that promote tissue building: insulin, insulinlike growth factors, testosterone, and growth hormone. Catabolic hormones, such as cortisol and progesterone, degrade cell proteins and inhibit tissue building.

Potentially the most powerful natural growth hormone stimulator known to science, exercise, is an unmatched anti-aging force, fat burner, and immune booster. It has the ability to unleash powerful hormonal forces within the body, which can be both beneficial and detrimental. For example, excessive reliance on aerobic exercise can suppress growth hormone and testosterone levels, rendering any amount of mass building impossible. It can also cause a catabolic outbreak, unleashing cortisol and other hostile catabolic hormones to assault the immune system, eating away at precious muscle tissue, and wreaking havoc within the body. On the other hand, anaerobic exercise can suppress the catabolic hormone cortisol and send testosterone and growth hormone levels soaring (in men), increasing sex drive, improving the ability to gain muscle mass, and opening the door to all the physiological and psychological benefits of youth. This is why many competitive bodybuilders limit aerobic activity during the muscle-building phase of their training to no more than 2 to 3 aerobic sessions per week for a maximum of 20 minutes each.

Testosterone

Testosterone is the primary androgen found in the body and is synthesized by cells in the testes, ovaries, and adrenal cortex. It is clear that testosterone directly affects the growth of skeletal muscle tissue, although not as much as

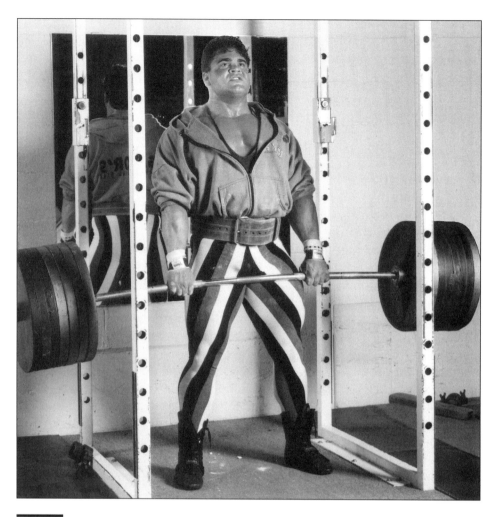

Strength training stimulates the hormones to maximize muscle-building potential.

growth hormone or insulinlike growth factors. Vigorous exercise stimulates the production of testosterone, as shown by increased testosterone levels in both athletes and nonathletes following moderate to heavy resistance workouts. The greatest change in serum testosterone levels seems to take place after regular involvement in resistance exercise for more than two years. The exercises that seem to play the greatest role in increasing testosterone concentrations target large-muscle groups (such as dead lifts and squats) and involve heavy resistance (85 to 95 percent of 1RM), multiple sets and / or multiple exercises, and rest intervals of 30 seconds to 1 minute.

Insulinlike Growth Factors

Insulinlike growth factors (IGFs) resemble insulin but do not react with insulin antibodies. IGFs are dependent on growth hormones and possess all the growth-promoting properties of the somatomedins. The response of IGFs is still largely unknown, but there is increasing evidence that the combined effects of growth hormone and IGFs are most responsible for the protein synthesis that leads to muscle growth. Growth hormone stimulates the production of IGFs in the cells of the muscle tissue, causing them to grow and possibly multiply (hyperplasia).

Growth Hormone

Growth hormone is critical for tissue repair, brain function, muscle growth, bone strength, and energy. This is accomplished by increasing circulating concentrations of free fatty acids, inhibiting the glucose absorption by peripheral tissues, and conserving blood glucose. Growth hormone does have some independent abilities in inducing growth in bone and muscles, but the primary role of growth hormone is to stimulate the production of IGFs, which are most responsible for muscle and bone growth. Other growth hormone functions include protein synthesis, fatty acid utilization, fat breakdown, glucose and amino acid release, and bone and cartilage growth.[4]

In every animal species, including humans, growth hormone declines with age. In humans over the age of 30, the amount of growth hormone drops about 22 percent every 10 years. By about the age of 65 growth hormone production is approximately 25 percent of its highest level at the age of 30. This pattern of decline is consistent with other anabolic hormones as well, such as testosterone and IGF. A number of conditions are affected, either directly or indirectly, by the decline in growth hormone, including

- muscle atrophy,
- decreased energy,
- increased abdominal fat,
- weak bones,
- reduced cardiac capacity,
- thinning skin and wrinkles,
- ineffective cognitive functioning,
- mood changes,
- reduced sexual performance, and
- impaired kidney function.

If growth hormone is so valuable, is it possible to slow the decline of growth hormone production? Absolutely. Growth hormone can be increased through prescription human growth hormone (HGH) injections, nutritional hormone stimulation, and resistance exercise. HGH injections, approved for use by adults in 1996 by the U.S. Federal Drug Administration, are available only by prescription and are rarely prescribed due to the high cost and specific purpose for which they are intended. Nutritional hormone stimulation, which increases HGH, involves stimulation of the hypothalamus and anterior pituitary to produce more HGH through amino acid stacking. Nutritional hormonal stimulation requires no prescription, has fewer potential side effects than HGH injections, and is relatively inexpensive. A greater discussion on the role of nutritional supplements in the life of a bodybuilder will be discussed in chapter 4.

The response of growth hormone to resistance training has not been extensively studied, but some evidence suggests that training will produce some change in immediate levels of growth hormone. These changes are most often associated with moderately heavy resistance exercise, although not all resistance exercise elicits the same response. The most dramatic serum increases in growth hormone take place under conditions of heavy resistance (less than 10 RM), with high volume (three or more sets), and with short rest periods between sets (60 seconds or less). Not everything is known about stimulating growth hormone production through exercise, certainly, but it is clear that the simplest and most cost effective method for stimulating growth hormone production is resistance exercise. It is up to individual bodybuilders to see that their programs are designed to ensure the optimal stimulation of muscle-building hormones release.

Cortisol

Cortisol has gotten a bad reputation among bodybuilders. Most are convinced that cortisol robs the body of hard-earned muscle and thus needs to be suppressed. Many bodybuilders will even take supplements in the hope that they will be able to suppress cortisol secretion and maintain muscle size and strength. The problem is, cortisol is necessary for many metabolic reactions in the body. At best, insufficient levels of cortisol could lead to muscle weakness. At worst, cortisol depletion could lead to death.

The purpose of cortisol is to break down large molecules into smaller molecules, called "catabolism." When you lift weights, cortisol is released to break the body proteins into amino acids, thus increasing the amino acid level in the blood. These amino acids then travel to the muscle fibers being stressed through exercise. The amino acids are reassembled into proteins that help repair damaged muscle fibers. Clearly, then, artificially reduced cortisol levels can mean sore muscles and even delayed muscle recovery after a workout.

The other primary advantages of cortisol are (1) it breaks down adipose tissue, and (2) even though it can break down proteins in the muscle, it does so in a preferential pattern. That is, cortisol does not appear to break down the functional proteins of the muscle. The answer to the cortisol question seems to be balance. Rather than suppress it, regulate it for optimal muscle rejuvenation. Eating and training intelligently, including avoiding extreme low-calorie diets and overtraining, seem to be the keys to counterbalance the negative effects of cortisol.[5]

Catecholamines

Epinephrine, norepinephrine, and dopamine make up the catecholamine family of hormones. While their role in muscle growth is unclear, it does seem that catecholamines augment the production of those hormones responsible for muscle growth, namely, testosterone, IGFs, and growth hormone. They also seem to play a direct role in the increase of force production, muscle contraction rate, and available energy, which suggests—if not proves—that they are probably one of the first neuroendocrine responses to resistance training.

The human machine is intricate, complex, and efficient. It is amazing what the human body is capable of doing when the mind and body work as one. It is capable of running at almost 30 mph, jumping more than 8 feet high and 30 feet long, and squatting more than 1,000 pounds. When your mind and body work together there is almost no limit on what you can achieve in the sport of bodybuilding. So, take care of your body and your mind and discover the power of the mind-body connection.

CHAPTER 4

Feeding the Muscles and Mind

Food is one of life's great pleasures. In fact, most holidays and social occasions, from Christmas to Thanksgiving to Easter, are centered on food. But food is much more than a backdrop for gatherings and conversation in social circles. Food provides nutrition for the body and the necessary energy to sustain quality of life. Sure, everyone knows that, but how does it happen? What are food allergies, and why do so many people struggle with eating disorders and obesity? Why are there so many different diets endorsed by doctors and so-called experts? And why is it that so many bodybuilders find nutrition and supplementation the most challenging part of the bodybuilding lifestyle? The problem is, most people, including bodybuilders, know just enough about nutrition to make themselves dangerous but not enough to get the full benefits of food and nutritional supplements.

Over the past 20 years, interest in nutrition and behavior has exploded, largely sparked by a corresponding interest in improving fitness and health. But while most people are eating healthier today than in the past, they still fail to understand the role of nutrition in enhancing physical and emotional well-being. The fact is, what you eat is just as important as getting enough sleep or having good workouts.

As its title suggests, this chapter focuses on feeding the mind and the muscles with food and supplements, offering specifics on how various foods and nutritional supplements can have a significant impact on mental and physical function, and behavior. Among the topics are the relationship between food and bodybuilding success; dysfunctional eating patterns and disorders; healthy eating patterns; eating for peak performance, including periodization; eating for strength and hypertrophy; and the use of supplements and drugs.

Bioenergetics

It seems obvious that conditioning programs should be specifically tailored for every athlete. Endurance athletes should follow training programs designed to improve the aerobic system, whereas athletes involved in power sports or activities will benefit most from anaerobic training programs. But what about nutrition? Should all athletes follow the same nutritional regimen? Clearly, it would make more sense for different athletes to follow specific nutritional programs. Amazingly, sport researchers have only recently begun to recognize the importance of specific nutritional practices for different types of exercise.

All living things, including bodybuilders, require a continual supply of energy in order to function. Energy is used for every process that keeps the body alive. Some of these processes are continual, such as the metabolism of foods, the synthesis of molecules like proteins and DNA, and the transport of molecules and ions through the body. Other processes, such as muscle contraction and certain cellular movements, occur only at certain times. Whatever the energy-requiring process, however, before energy can be used, it must first be transformed into a form the organism can easily handle.

Adenosine triphosphate (ATP) is the molecule that carries energy. Made up of three phosphate groups, ATP works by losing the endmost phosphate group when instructed to do so by an enzyme. This reaction, which produces adenosine diphosphate (ADP), releases a lot of energy, which the body then uses to build proteins and contract muscles. Still more energy can be extracted by removing a second phosphate group, producing adenosine monophosphate (AMP). When the muscles are at rest and energy is not needed, the reverse reaction takes place. Each phosphate group is reattached to the molecule using energy obtained from food or sunlight. ATP is like a tree trunk. It stores energy and is able to release it when needed.

Because the only substance that can be used for skeletal contraction is ATP, the phosphate groups liberated from ATP must be continually replaced to allow ongoing energy transfer. It is interesting to note that the reactions of ATP usually require hydrolysis, meaning that ATP will be most effective if the body is adequately hydrated. When muscular fatigue causes the skeletal contraction exercise (i.e., weight training) to terminate, it is often because the intensity was too high to maintain a steady state and ATP regeneration was not possible.

ATP is positively related to muscle mass. In other words, the greater the muscle mass, the greater the ATP stores. Enhancement of ATP stores over and above that which is expected, given the amount of muscle mass, is not supported by research and tends to be quite controversial. Where there seems to be little controversy is in the role that another metabolic molecule, creatine phosphate (CP), plays in delivering energy to working muscles.

CP exceeds ATP concentrations by approximately five times. CP contains only one phosphate group, but it is capable of donating its phosphate immediately to support the regeneration of ADP to ATP, as discussed earlier. When activity begins, metabolic balance in the body cannot be maintained and CP stores of phosphate are immediately mobilized. The higher the intensity of the exercise, the more rapidly the stores will become depleted. The greater the initial level of CP, the longer it takes for the stores to be depleted. This is the basis for creatine monohydrate supplementation. Creatine monohydrate, a popular supplement among bodybuilders, is designed to maximize the store of CP.

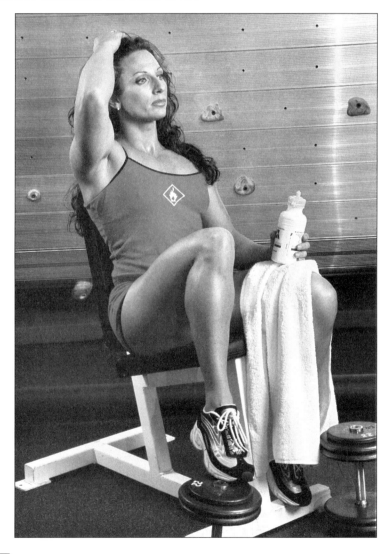

A nutritional break during a workout provides you with the energy you need.

Although CP is the immediate source of phosphates to transform ADP to ATP, this essential reaction cannot replenish the system effectively until the activity has subdued. This is why the rest interval between sets is so important for bodybuilders. The rest interval gives CP the opportunity to supply the muscles with energy needed for each successive set. Bodybuilders who have adequate stores of CP and allow sufficient time for ATP regeneration will experience great muscle growth.

Food and Bodybuilding

Next to an effective training program, proper nutrition is probably the most important factor in achieving bodybuilding success. In fact, some bodybuilders are convinced that nutritional supplementation is even more important than a solid training program. No matter the order of importance, the body needs nutrients to build solid muscle mass. This includes the proper balance of carbohydrates, fats, and proteins, as well as the appropriate caloric balance to gain muscle, cut body fat, or both. Of course, good nutrition is also essential for muscle growth and repair, maintenance, and enough energy to sustain the bodybuilding lifestyle. It is simply not possible for bodybuilders to take full advantage of their training if they are not getting an adequate supply of nutrients.

It is important to remember that your body is incredibly resilient. You can feed it whatever "garbage" you want and it will most likely survive, at least in the short term. But bodybuilding is not about surviving. Bodybuilding is about going beyond everyday expectations for health and well-being. The bodybuilder who wants a hard-packed, muscular physique must plan to go beyond the average and strive to reach the highest level of health. Your body does not consider muscle mass essential for survival. To build muscle mass, you will need to approach nutrition with the same scientific fortitude that you use in physical training. That will necessitate learning how to provide your body with the proper nutrients it needs to carry out the muscle-building process.

Many excellent books outline the nutritional requirements for recreational and competitive bodybuilding. Many cover the optimal balance of nutrients, proper caloric intake, and ideal timing of meals. This chapter is not intended as a thorough examination of nutrition but rather as a study of the mind-body connection in relation to food, specifically the positive or negative influence food can have on the success of a bodybuilder.

Have you ever noticed all the different ways athletes eat? Some people eat three square meals a day; some skip breakfast and then eat a large lunch and dinner; some eat a small breakfast, a large lunch, and a small dinner; and so on. It is no different in the bodybuilding world. Bodybuilders have unique and diverse eating patterns. Some bodybuilders eat three large meals a day and snack between those meals on protein bars and shakes, while other bodybuilders eat as many as eight meals and consume as much as 10,000 calories a day. There are almost as many different eating patterns as there are bodybuilders.

Complete exercise 4.1 to determine if you have any dysfunctional eating patterns that could interfere with optimal muscle growth and fitness. Then compare your eating habits with those explained in the next section to identify your patterns.

Exercise 4.1   Eating Patterns Analysis

1. How many times per day do you eat a meal? A meal is any amount of food that is intended to give you the feeling of being satisfied and would likely be more than 1,000 calories. _____

2. Explain your reasons for eating that number of meals each day. For example, you may need to eat as much as possible to gain muscular size.

   _____

   _____

3. How many times per day do you snack? A snack is any amount of food that partially satisfies you, typically less than 500 calories. _____

4. Explain the reasons you have for eating that number of snacks each day. For example, you may believe that the only way you can consume an adequate volume of food is by eating plenty of snacks each day.

   _____

   _____

5. Do you know the approximate percentage of carbohydrates, proteins, and fats that you consume in your diet each day? If you do, list them here.

   _____

6. Check off which, if any, of the eating pattern behaviors below are characteristic of your eating behaviors:
   - Intentionally skipping breakfast or other meals
   - Eating large volumes of a single food source such as beef, chicken, or pasta
   - Staying completely away from a single food source because of something that you "heard" about it
   - Changing diet plans every time you read a new book or magazine article on nutrition

(continued)

- Eating large amounts of food when not feeling physically hungry
- Supplanting meals with commercially prepared meal replacements
- Thinking about food throughout the day to the point of becoming obsessed with it
- Spending enormous amounts of time each day in preparing and ingesting food
- Measuring every meal to determine if it has "adequate" caloric qualities and the "appropriate" balance of nutrients
- Attempting to eliminate all fat from your diet
- Only buying food that is labelled "calorie reduced," "fat free," and "suitable for diets"
- Craving certain foods such as chocolate, ice cream, or potato chips
- Eating large volumes of food in one sitting and then going the rest of the day (or many days) eating very little
- Strictly adhering to a specific diet plan (i.e., The Zone, Carbohydrate Addicts Diet, Pritikin Promise)

7. For any of the eating pattern behaviours that you checked off in Question 6, indicate why it is that you engage in that behavior including any research that you may have done to encourage you in that behavior.

_____

_____

_____

_____

_____

_____

8. Using the scale below, circle the number that best corresponds with how satisfied you are with your current eating pattern.

1	2	3	4	5	6
Completely dissatisfied	Moderately dissatisfied	Somewhat dissatisfied	Somewhat satisfied	Moderately satisfied	Completely satisfied

9. What things must you do to become more satisfied with your current eating patterns?

_____

_____

10. Are you satisfied that you have sufficient knowledge of appropriate eating patterns for bodybuilding success? If the answer is no, then what must you do to get that knowledge?

    _____

    _____

11. Using the scale below, circle the number that best corresponds with the level of support that you have from family and significant others to establish good eating patterns (i.e., grocery purchasing, meal preparation, flexibility in meal times).

1	2	3	4	5	6
Not support	Very Little support	Some support	Moderate support	Much support	Complete support

12. Indicate the types of support that you have from family and significant others in establishing and maintaining good eating patterns. What are some other types of support that would make things easier for you?

    _____

    _____

    _____

    _____

Dysfunctional Eating Patterns

Like all athletes, bodybuilders must have both a long-term commitment to a physical training routine and the ability to overcome many emotional and mental challenges. Unlike other sports, however, success in bodybuilding has little to do with athletic prowess and strategy, and more to do with body size, symmetry, and definition. Indeed, no other sport bases success on looks rather than performance. As a result, probably no athletes are more preoccupied with food and nutritional supplementation than bodybuilders.

Since the early 1960s, there has been enough scientific research on athletic nutrition to fill a small library. Yet many bodybuilders continue to engage in dysfunctional eating patterns. Unhealthy eating does nothing to help bodybuilders develop a muscular frame, and in many cases, may actually destroy muscle tissue. You would think that bodybuilders would avoid eating patterns that destroy muscle tissue, but the story of Bill and Bob and the chicken egg may shed light on how this happens.

Once there were two brothers, Bill and Bob. Bill knew all about eggs being an excellent source of protein, but had never heard that they were high in cholesterol. The opposite was true of Bob. He knew that eggs were high in cholesterol, but had never heard that they were a good source of protein. To get large quantities of the protein essential for proper body functioning and muscular development, Bill decided that he would eat a dozen eggs every morning for breakfast. It only made sense, he figured. If they are so good for you, then you should eat lots of them! Bob, on the other hand, knowing that too much cholesterol is bad for the heart and arteries, decided that he would cut eggs out of his diet completely. "Why eat eggs if they are only going to kill you?" he figured.

This story is overly simplistic, but you can see the problem. Each brother simply based his eating patterns on one small piece of information. Many dysfunctional eating patterns start just that way. Consider the number of people currently cutting all fat from their diets. They know that ingesting too much fat is unhealthy, so they cut it out completely. The problem is, they are focusing on just one piece in the puzzle. Fat provides a concentrated form of energy and gives food a high satiety value. Fat also serves as a carrier of fat-soluble vitamins A, D, E, and K. Without fat, these vitamins quickly pass though the body. Finally, fat assists in the formation of muscle tissue, which helps us retain heat. To be sure, many people eat a diet that is far too high in fat to be healthy—too many, in fact. Nevertheless, having no fat in the diet can be just as harmful.

Look at table 4.1 and see if you or anyone you know can relate to any of the behavior changes that stem from true but small pieces of information.

Sooner or later, most bodybuilders stop eating the way they should. They may skip meals, decreasing their energy level and muscle growth potential while at the same time accumulating body fat. Others may live on "diet" foods but consume such large quantities that they end up fat anyway. Still others cycle on and off diets, eating compulsively or bingeing on high-fat treats.

These eating patterns can be harmful enough on their own, but they can also be warning signs of potentially serious eating disorders that should not be ignored. This book outlines the symptoms and harmful side effects of eating disorders, but if you suspect that you or someone you know has an eating disorder (for example, anorexia nervosa and bulimia nervosa), you should seek medical advice as soon as possible. Following is a list of dysfunctional eating patterns most common to intermediate and advanced bodybuilders.

Binge Eating

Binge eating refers to rapidly consuming abnormally large amounts of food in a relatively short period of time. It does not refer to those of us (myself included) who a few times per year (Christmas, Thanksgiving, and so on) eat such large volumes of food that it hurts to move. Binge eating often occurs in compulsive eaters, a category many bodybuilders fall into. Because they

Table 4.1   "One Fact" Diets

Fact	Behavior
Eggs are an excellent source of protein.	Eat as many eggs as possible at breakfast.
Eggs are high in cholesterol.	Cut eggs out of the diet completely.
Eating fat is bad for you.	Cut out fat completely.
Meat and dairy products are high in fat.	Become a vegan (one who cuts out all meat, cheese, and eggs).
Protein is essential for optimal bone and muscle development.	Eat copious amounts of protein, regardless of fat intake or stress on the kidneys.
The accumulation of body fat comes from ingesting more calories than are expended each day.	Cut out breakfast to reduce caloric intake.
One pound of fat contains approximately 3,500 calories.	Severely restrict daily caloric intake to lose weight quickly.
Vitamins and minerals are essential for health and well-being.	Rely on vitamin and mineral supplements, as opposed to healthy eating and exercise.

must eat enough food to build muscle, yet keep the total number of calories and dietary fat intake in check, it is not uncommon for bodybuilders to be become obsessed with food. In some cases, this obsession with a muscle-building diet spins out of control, to the point that bodybuilders severely restrict themselves at home, work, and in social settings. The pressure to cheat on a strict diet simply becomes too great. And once a crack appears in their willpower armor, binge eating begins.

Not only is the number of calories consumed very high (as much as 5,000 calories in one sitting!), but binge eating is also often dominated by foods that were restricted on the original diet, such as snack foods, alcohol, and other foods with little (if any) nutritional value and high fat content.

Ben, a bodybuilding friend, regularly binged to help him cope with dietary restrictions. Ben would adhere to his low-fat diet for a full week or two, consuming no alcohol, desserts, snack foods, or anything of the sort.

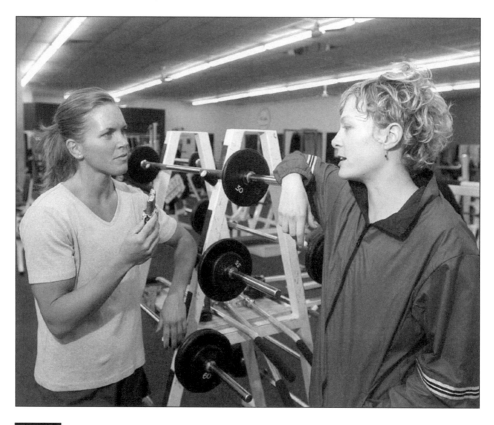

Proper nutrition is easier when you have good social support.

Basically, any food that did not play a significant role in muscle growth was prohibited. This was difficult for him, because he really enjoyed getting together with friends for meals and drinks on the weekends, but he believed that cutting them out was the only way he would be able to develop the body he wanted. It was not long before these severe food restrictions became too difficult to maintain, and Ben would start to binge.

Like figure 4.1 illustrates, after bingeing on high-fat foods and/or alcohol, he would feel so guilty that he vowed never to binge again. To make sure, Ben would restrict his diet more severely to make up for his latest indulgence and recommit himself to his dietary program. Again and again, the more restrictions he placed on his diet, the more he would feel pressure to cheat. You see, as the cycle of bingeing escalates, self-confidence wanes and feelings of helplessness begin to creep in.

It has been estimated that as many as 2 percent of North Americans are binge eaters. I would venture to guess that this percentage is higher among bodybuilders, simply because bodybuilders are so concerned with diet and body image. To be considered a binge eater, three of the following symptoms have to be present:

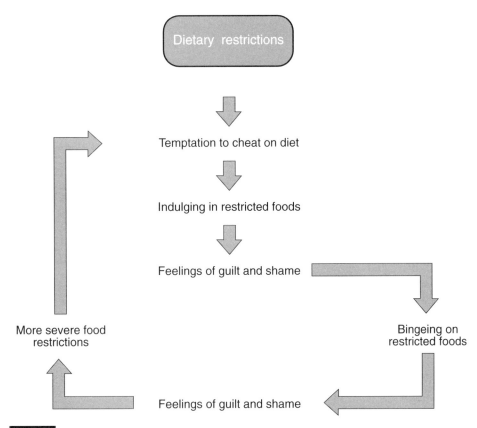

Figure 4.1 Bingeing cycle.

- Restricting your diet so severely that it is impossible to follow for any length of time
- Eating more rapidly than usual
- Eating to the point that you feel uncomfortable
- Eating large volumes of food when you are not hungry
- Eating large amounts of food throughout the day with no planned mealtimes
- Eating alone because you are embarrassed about how much food you consume and your eating habits

What can bodybuilders do to change a binge-eating pattern into a pattern more appropriate for muscle development? It is clear that one of the most obvious causes of binge eating among bodybuilders is severe dietary restrictions, so it only makes sense to start there. Why not relax a little on your diet? Why not allow yourself a treat every once in a while?

Because of the North American "fast food" mentality, we want things to come easily. We do not want to have to wait. And that includes the way we look. Our thinking goes something like this: "I want a ripped, muscular physique, and I know that high-fat foods do not contribute to my goal. Therefore, even though I love eating snack foods, I am going to cut them from my diet completely so that I can reach my goal as fast as possible."

What is the rush? Why not enjoy the process and smell the roses, so to speak? It is possible that it could take a little longer to get the body you want, but the changes will be permanent and the process will have been far more healthy and enjoyable.

The first thing to try if you are a binge eater is to eat smaller, more frequent meals. Determine the number of calories that you should be consuming each day and then divide that amount into three equal-sized meals and three smaller snacks. Eating smaller meals throughout the day is the best pattern for food digestion and weight management. If you find that you are unable to conquer the binge-eating pattern by eating smaller, more frequent meals and treating yourself every once in a while, you may need professional help to change the behavior. There is nothing wrong with asking for help. Moreover, if you truly want to improve your health and the way you look, you should be glad to have the help available. Treatment of severe binge eating usually includes education, various behavioral programs, and therapy.

Compulsive Overeating

It has always amazed me how many so-called bodybuilders just look fat. In their clothes, it is difficult to tell the difference between them and any obese person. They may have large muscles and be very strong, but there is nothing ripped and defined about their bodies. I had a student in my office a few years ago who told me that he was a bodybuilder and was interested in getting big. I did not have the heart to tell him that he was already big, although not in the way he desired. He had a large chest and very big arms, to be sure, but his waist was bigger than his chest. This student did not need to get bigger; he needed to lose body fat.

Many bodybuilders fail to understand that bodybuilding is not only about size and strength but about visible muscle growth as well. A linebacker may find it advantageous to have a large muscular frame hidden under a layer of adipose tissue, much as a sumo wrestler and power lifter would, but it is not the case in bodybuilding. Too often, bodybuilders become severely obese because they function under another "one fact" truth: to get muscular, you must consume large volumes of food. This is partially true. Building muscle does require additional calories, but not nearly as many as some bodybuilders think.

Assuming your current diet is adequate to maintain your body weight, you probably already know that gaining 1 pound requires 3,500 additional calories. You may also know that, for well-trained male athletes, the maximum amount of muscle you can gain in a month is approximately 1.5 pounds per month, or 18 pounds per year. (For untrained men, muscle gain in the

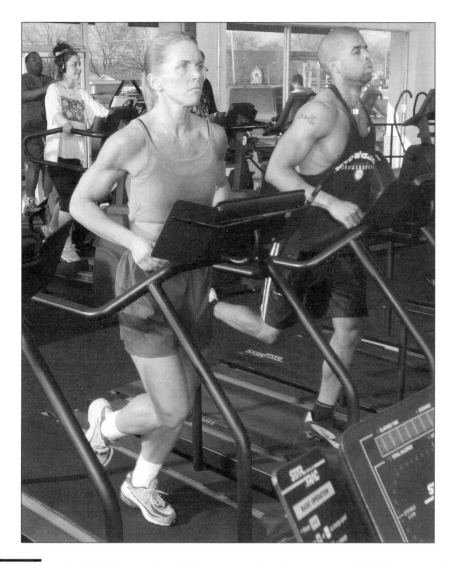

Women require half the total caloric consumption increase required by men when gaining 8 to 10 pounds of muscle.

first year can be as much as 25 pounds.) Female athletes can expect to gain 8 to 12 pounds of muscle per year. If a trained bodybuilder wanting to gain 18 pounds of muscle in a year were to maintain his current lifestyle and activity levels, he would need to increase total caloric consumption during the year by approximately 63,000 calories, or 172.3 calories per day (not accounting for changes in basal metabolism due to increased muscle mass). This is equivalent to 1 breast of chicken, 2 soft-boiled eggs, or 3 ounces of roast beef per day, in addition to all other food intake. Females interested in gaining 8 to 10 pounds of muscle, would need to increase total caloric consumption during the year by approximately half of the increase required for the male bodybuilder.

An untrained individual wanting to gain 18 pounds of muscle would have to consume the same 63,000 additional calories, plus another 66,500 to cover the caloric expenditure of the added weight-training workouts (175-pound man, 4 one-hour workouts per week, 50 weeks per year). This means that for an untrained man to gain 18 pounds of muscle in one year, he would have to begin working out with weights four times per week and consume an additional 354.8 calories per day (not accounting for changes in basal metabolism due to increased muscle mass).

Thus, rather than make small increases in caloric consumption during the day, many bodybuilders become compulsive overeaters who simply cannot stop putting food into their mouths. They eat fast; they eat a lot; they even eat when they are full; they may also eat around the clock—all in the name of gaining muscle. Contrary to popular belief, it is not necessary to get fat in the off-season to gain muscle for competition. The truth is, the 500 to 1,000 additional daily calories that many novice bodybuilders ingest will help them gain much more than just the 18 to 25 pounds of muscle they desire, but much of that additional weight will be fat. Along with the added muscle, a bodybuilder eating 500 to 1,000 additional calories per day can expect to gain somewhere between 15 and 50 pounds of fat in one year.

It can be difficult to find the perfect balance of caloric intake that will ensure optimal muscle growth without adding unwanted body fat. Since gaining muscle is not an exact science it would be better to gain some fat in the off-season and know that optimal muscle growth occurred rather than the opposite. The problem is that too many bodybuilders gain too much fat in the off-season and find that shedding it can be incredibly burdensome. I believe that the "6 percent rule" is a good guide. That is, body fat loss from the off-season to the competitive season should be no more than 6 percent of your total weight. For example, if you have an off-season weight of 240 pounds, then your ripped, competitive weight should be no less than 225.6 pounds. Stated another way, if you had more than 14.4 pounds to lose before competition, then you would have too much body fat in the off-season.

The following symptoms are characteristic of compulsive overeaters.

- Turning to food when depressed, lonely, rejected, or in need of a reward
- Believing that eating large volumes of food, regardless of nutritional value, is necessary for muscle growth
- Constantly thinking and talking about food throughout the day
- Eating quickly without enjoyment and continuing to eat after hunger has been satisfied

To stop eating compulsively, educate yourself about the true caloric needs to gain muscle; eat more slowly; plan as many as six moderate meals per day, each emphasizing proper nutritional balance; avoid eating between meals; and stop eating when you are no longer hungry. Do not fool yourself by

Nutritional Spotlight: Lena Johannesen

Lena Johannesen is an IFBB fitness professional and international fitness model. She has competed in many different fitness competitions, including the Ms. Fitness International (1997-2000) and Ms. Fitness Olympia (1997-2000) contests. As one of the most sought-after fitness models in the world, she has been on more than 15 magazine covers, including *Muscle & Fitness* and *Flex*. You can learn more about Lena by checking out her website (**http://www.lenajohannesen.com**). Here are some of her thoughts on proper nutrition and diet:

As one of the world's top fitness competitors and models, I've been through trial and error when it comes to diet and nutrition, including what to eat, when to eat, and so on. The one thing I could always count on was that good nutrition was necessary to create the body I could be happy with. I could train and train, but if I did not provide my body with the right fuel to get through the grueling workouts, I never saw any real results.

If you have goals for your physical training, the nutrition part is easier. Start out easy with small goals, such as going a full month without missing a workout or improving your bench press by 20 pounds. Then you can move up to larger challenges, such as entering a competition, losing 2 to 3 inches on your waistline, and losing 10 percent of your body fat This way you can see how your body reacts before tackling larger challenges.

I think that the most difficult part of staying committed is during holidays and weekends, when I get bored or I'm out partying with friends, and late nights are common. I have found, however, that there are always alternatives when eating out. For example, rather than order a burger and fries with a Coke, go for a chicken salad (or rice) with a Diet Coke. It is that simple, and it tastes great. To overcome the late-night cravings, eat some fresh-cut vegetables like carrots, celery, and cauliflower. Nibble on them when the cravings hit during the day as well. Diet soda, protein shakes, and a piece of chicken breast are also good alternatives.

In the end, we are only human. I believe that we should enjoy life and have fun with friends from time to time. I know that most competitive athletes (myself included) allow themselves a "cheat day" or at least a "cheat meal" once a week. I think that's good. In fact, cheating once in a while can make the whole diet process much easier. Not only does it give you something to look forward to, but "shocking" your body with different foods can actually speed up your metabolism. So allow yourself a treat now and then, but make sure you get back on track the very next day.

believing that being fat for a good part of the year is a necessary part of the bodybuilding lifestyle.

Extreme Dieting

Bodybuilders use extreme diets to lose large amounts of body fat and get ripped before a competition or the beach season. As with compulsive overeating or carrying large amounts of adipose tissue during the off-season, the difficulty with extreme dieting is that it causes more harm than good. Extreme dieting causes serious vitamin and mineral deficiencies, decreased bone size and strength, lack of energy and motivational drive, and decreased muscle strength and size.

Have you ever heard that dieting makes you fat? Yes, it makes you fat! You have likely seen people who seem to eat like birds yet never seem to lose weight. Why is that? Well, their basal metabolic rate (BMR) is so low that almost no level of caloric consumption would be low enough for them to lose weight.

BMR is the rate you burn calories while at rest. In other words, the faster your BMR, the more calories your body requires to maintain normal function throughout the day, including during sleep. BMR is relatively constant, cannot be changed quickly, and is largely influenced by genetic factors. Research shows that BMR is affected by gender and age, with males and younger adults having the fastest BMRs. This is why teenage boys and young adult males seem to be able to eat anything they want and not gain weight. If you are a female or getting older, you will just have to put up with a lower BMR and thus lower caloric demands.

Does this sound fatalistic? Well, there is some good news. BMR is also affected by body size, bone thickness, and muscular size. In other words, the more muscle you have, the higher your BMR!

So what does extreme dieting have to do with bodybuilding? BMR is negatively affected by severe caloric restrictions. When the body lacks sufficient calories to function normally, it begins to shut down nonessential functions. It goes into survival mode. While you may believe that gaining muscle size and strength are part of normal function, your body does not. In fact, when your body goes into survival mode, it begins to eat away at the hard-packed muscle you worked so hard to develop, using it as survival fuel.

Extreme dieters often think they know a great deal about nutrition, but as with compulsive overeaters and binge eaters, their knowledge is usually based on misconceptions or misguided beliefs. The following symptoms are characteristic of extreme dieting.

- Overriding compulsion to be thin or ripped
- Severe reduction in caloric intake, sometimes to less than 1,000 calories per day

- Constantly excited about the latest diet
- Reliance on a limited selection of foods (such as the infamous "grape-fruit diet")

Most bodybuilders are able to change the harmful pattern of extreme dieting simply by becoming more knowledgeable about their bodies and the role that nutrition plays in body composition. For some avid dieters, however, including those who deny that they have a problem, professional help in the form of counseling and/or medical treatment may be necessary.

Overconsumption of Protein

One of the most common eating disorders among bodybuilders is the overriding obsession with adequate protein intake. There is no doubt that protein is the basic nutrient required for building muscle tissue. The problem is simply "too much of a good thing." Just as too many eggs can cause an increase in low-density cholesterol, so can the ingestion of too much protein be harmful. While it is true that bodybuilders and other strength athletes require more protein than sedentary individuals, bodybuilders do not require as much as they often think.

The average sedentary person requires approximately .36 grams of protein for every pound of body weight. Research on nutrition in endurance and strength sports reveals that endurance athletes require approximately .60 grams of protein for every pound of body weight, while strength athletes need .72 grams. In other words, the bodybuilder needs approximately twice as much protein as the sedentary individual and 20 percent more than an endurance athlete.

Since most of the additional protein required for bodybuilding will come from an increase in food consumption, significant protein supplementation is both unnecessary and potentially dangerous. Excess protein is sometimes burned as fuel, and a highly inefficient form of fuel at that. More likely, however, excess protein is stored as fat. Overconsumption of protein can also lead to such health problems as dehydration, kidney damage, and ketosis. There is a place for protein supplementation in the bodybuilding lifestyle, certainly, but it should be used with caution.

If, after reading this, you are still concerned that you are not getting enough protein to support optimal muscle growth, you may find it helpful to begin a program of protein supplementation. Your body can easily handle as much as 1 gram of protein per pound of body weight without danger. However, while there is plenty of research to support the negative side effects associated with excessive protein intake, there is no scientific research to support ingesting more than 1 gram per pound of body weight (including food and supplement consumption). So be sure that protein supplementation does not take you beyond the optimal level for both health and muscle growth.

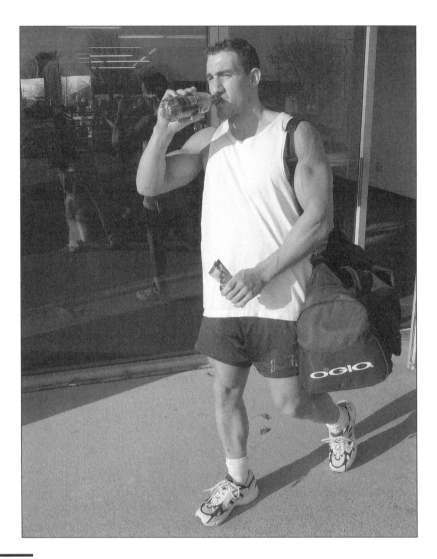

Nutrition after a workout is important to replenish the exhausted muscles.

Eating Periodization

Have you ever heard of the law of supply and demand? It is a law in economics that states that price is determined by the supply of a product and consumer demand for that product. It goes on to state that the supply of goods will always attempt to meet the demands of the consumer. This is exactly the way that the body functions. To stimulate muscle growth, you need to place enough demand (stress) on your muscles to create an adaptive response. This enables the muscles to supply greater force during the next workout, and over time the muscles simply grow larger as they adapt to the stress.

For this adaptation to occur at an optimal level, your diet must supply the nutritional components necessary for muscular growth. If your diet is poor, you can forget about gaining size. If your diet is excessively high in calories and/or fat, you can count on layers of body fat being added to your muscular frame. Just as your training program will change over the course of a year (cycling your training is discussed in chapter 8), so should your nutritional program. In fact, your nutrition program should match the training goals you set for each period. This is called *eating periodization.*

Table 4.2 gives you an indication of how to connect your nutrition and training programs. If, for example, your goal is to increase muscle mass, look under the "Hypertrophy" column. If you simply want to increase muscle strength, look under the "Strength" column. If you want to increase power, which is a combination of muscle strength and speed required of powerlifters in competition, look under the "Power" column. And so on.

As table 4.2 shows, your training goals also determine the type of supplementation you need to reach peak performance. Research shows that creatine and glutamine are best for individuals wanting to increase muscle strength, power, and size. Creatine is primarily used to increase muscle power, strength, and recovery from difficult training sets. It also leads to an increase in body weight, partially because of water retention. Glutamine helps to prevent muscle breakdown and to support the immune system while in heavy periods of training.

Many bodybuilders believe that if a supplement is good for them, they can increase the benefit by taking more. In fact, more is not better when it comes to most supplements. Recommended doses of creatine range from 2 to 20 milligrams, but current research shows that 3 to 8 milligrams of creatine per day is most effective. Bodybuilders should take 5 to 20 milligrams of glutamine per day.

Other supplements that may be effective for enhancing muscle growth include branched-chain amino acids (BCAAs), alanine, and taurine, but scientific support for them is mostly anecdotal evidence and inconclusive research. Individuals wanting to enhance fat loss may find benefit in ingesting caffeine (100 to 300 milligrams per day) to promote fat utilization and ephedrine (20 to 75 milligrams per day) to raise metabolism and increase fat mobilization.

While nutritional supplements can sometimes take a bodybuilder over the edge of a training plateau or static growth, many of the supplements endorsed in bodybuilding magazines are at best ineffective and at worst harmful. Do not waste your hard-earned money on supplements that will just end up being "flushed" away. For more information on nutritional supplementation for bodybuilders, peruse some well-regarded books on nutrition. You may also find it helpful to read some of the scientific research published in bodybuilding magazines, such as *Muscle & Fitness* magazine's annual nutrition issue published every March.

Table 4.2 Nutrition and Training Periodization

Goal	Hypertrophy	Strength	Power	Fat loss and muscle maintenance	Optimal looks and competition	Recuperation and renewal
Nutrition plan	• Add 500-1,000 for men; 250-500 for women; calories per day to daily intake. • Consume 1g of protein per lb of body weight. • Consume 3:1 ratio of carbohydrates to protein. • Approximately 20% of diet should be fat. • Eat 4-5 meals per day. • Supplement diet with meal replacement	• Add 500-1,000 for men; 250-500 for women; calories per day to daily intake. • Consume 1g of protein per lb of body weight. • Consume 3:1 ratio of carbohydrates to protein. • Approximately 20% of diet should be fat. • Eat 4-5 meals per day. • Supplement diet with meal replacement	• Add 500-1,000 for men; 250-500 for women; calories per day to daily intake. • Consume 1g of protein per lb of body weight. • Consume 3:1 ratio of carbohydrates to protein. • Approximately 20% of diet should be fat. • Eat 4-5 meals per day. • Supplement diet with meal replacement	• Decrease your current caloric intake by 500-1,000 calories per day. • Consume 1g of protein per lb of body weight. • Consume 2:1 ratio of carbohydrates to protein. • Approximately 15% of diet should be fat. • Eat 3-4 meals per day. • Take whey protein, caffeine, and ephedrine once per day.	• Stabilize caloric intake to a level where no weight is gained or lost. • Consume 1g of protein per lb of body weight. • Consume 2:1 ratio of carbohydrates to protein. • Approximately 15% of diet should be fat. • Eat 3-4 meals per day. • Take whey	• Take a break and have some fun. Keep the following points in mind, but feel free to eat whatever you want, whenever you want. • Consume 1g of protein per lb of body weight. • Consume 2:1 ratio of carbohydrates to protein. • Approximately 25% of diet should be fat. • Eat 3-4 meals per day. • Take a multivi-

	• shake once per day. • Take whey protein, creatine, and glutamine once per day. • Take a multivitamin/mineral supplement once per day.	• shake once per day. • Take whey protein, creatine, and glutamine once per day. • Take a multivitamin/mineral supplement once per day.	• shake once per day. • Take whey protein, creatine, and glutamine once per day. • Take a multivitamin/mineral supplement once per day.	• Take a multivitamin/mineral supplement once per day.	• protein, creatine, and ephedrine once per day. • Take a multivitamin/mineral supplement once per day.	tamin/mineral supplement once per day.
Type of training	• 4–5 weight workouts per week • 18–24 sets per workout • 3–5 sets per exercise • 8–12 reps per set • 50–75% of 1RM • 60–90 seconds rest between sets • 20–30 minutes aerobic training • 2–3 times per week	• 3–4 weight workouts per week • 14–18 sets per workout • 3–5 sets per exercise • 5–6 reps per set • 80–88% of 1RM • 90–150 seconds rest between sets • 15–20 minutes aerobic training • 2–3 times per week	• 3–4 weight workouts per week • 12–14 sets per workout • 3–5 sets per exercise • 2–4 reps per set • 90–95% of 1RM • 150–210 seconds rest between sets • 15–20 minutes aerobic training • 2–3 times per week	• 3–4 weight workouts per week • 16–20 sets per workout • 3–5 sets per exercise • 10–15 reps per set • 60–70% of 1RM • 45–75 seconds rest between sets • 30–45 minutes aerobic training • 4–5 times per week	• 4 weight workouts per week • 12–16 sets per workout • 2–4 sets per exercise • 8–12 reps per set • 65–80% of 1RM • 60–90 seconds rest between sets • 30–45 minutes aerobic training • 4–5 times per	• No more than 2, 30-minute, full-body workouts per week • Other activities such as hiking, swimming, cycling, and tennis

Building Naturally Versus Pharmacologically

To use or not to use, that is the question. At one time or another, most serious bodybuilders will have to make a decision about whether they are going to be a natural bodybuilder or a "chemical" bodybuilder. It seems like such an easy decision to say no to the use of performance-enhancing drugs, at least on the surface. You would have to have lived in the deep jungles of Africa since 1980 not to have heard about the negative side effects of using anabolic (tissue-building) steroids, growth hormone, or other muscle-enhancing drugs. Of course, if it is so easy to say no to performance-enhancing drugs, then why are so many elite athletes using them? Maybe, just maybe, it is not such an easy question. Perhaps it is not an easy choice for those bodybuilders who want to be the best. Perhaps there is no other way to create the optimal body.

In the 1970s, bodybuilders began to experiment with anabolic steroids. The more anabolic steroids they took, the closer they came to body perfection, both in shape and muscular size. The steroids were highly effective, and the resulting body changes became addictive. Public attention, desired by every bodybuilder, only served to further entrench the habit of chemically inducing physical change. Chemical bodybuilders were hungry to discover and consume newer and better anabolic agents, and the anabolic industry did not fail them.[1]

Pretty quickly, "chemical" bodybuilders found themselves moving from low-dose anabolic steroids to extremely large doses. They became psychologically and physiologically addicted to the drugs, because without them they could no longer maintain the physique they had grown to love. Initially they would cycle on and off the drugs to allow their bodies to recover, but this pattern soon faded in favor of a "continued use for continual growth" philosophy. Simply put, the effects of anabolic steroid use—enhanced muscle growth, positive changes in mood, an increased desire to train, and the ability to recover from intense exercise—promotes continued use. Because this psychological training boost is quickly dissipated when the steroids are discontinued, bodybuilders become addicted to using them.

It is important for you to understand that anabolic steroids and other forms of hormonal manipulation will, in fact, enhance training performance and appearance. They are designed to increase the constructive metabolic pathways within the body and make the body grow in ways that would not otherwise be possible. Anabolic steroids alter the body's hormonal balance, resulting in an enhancement of the anabolic properties of androgens (male hormones). Thus, without a strong commitment to an intensive strength-training program, positive effects of hormonal manipulation will be limited. Study after study has shown that the anabolic effects of both anabolic steroids and HGH are maximized when combined with intense exercise.

Bodybuilders who desire the optimal body will have to ask themselves whether the benefits outweigh the risks of using performance-enhancing drugs. Before making that decision for yourself, it would be wise to become informed. Understanding the physiological and psychological effects of prolonged anabolic steroid and HGH use is a good start.

Anabolic Steroids

Anabolic steroids are the most common drug used by competitive bodybuilders and strength athletes to gain a competitive edge. While they have shown themselves to be an effective change agent in promoting muscle growth, however, they are not without serious side effects.

Physiological Effects

Two general categories of physiological effects are associated with the use of anabolic steroids: anabolic and androgenic. Anabolic effects are desirable, of course, and although the greatest effects are seen in females and hypogonadal or castrated males, gains can also be seen in physiologically normal males. Anabolic steroids are meant to mimic the natural male sex hormone testosterone. The use of anabolic steroids increases fat-free weight gain, and muscle fiber is enlarged when steroids are used in conjunction with a strength-training program. Strength gain, which usually precedes size gain, can also be increased by steroid use. Interestingly enough, anabolic steroids only provide maximum benefit to highly trained athletes, such as bodybuilders, who add them to an existing training program.

So which is responsible for the muscular changes? The physiological effect of the steroid, or the euphoric moods that encourage more rigorous workouts? Research indicates that while there are definite psychological benefits to taking steroids, there are also substantial physiological benefits that cannot be obtained with a positive mind-set alone.

But before the steroid picture seems too rosy, here are the negatives. The undesirable side effects of taking steroids are the androgenic effects. These range from temporary or reversible changes to permanent and serious changes. For a list of the anabolic and androgenic changes attributed to anabolic steroids, see table 4.3.

Psychological Effects

While the research on the psychological effects of anabolic steroids is in its infant stages, it is clear that most bodybuilders and athletes who use anabolic steroids go through significant behavioral changes. Some even experience a complete personality change. Yes, some of those changes can be positive. It is hard to imagine any bodybuilder who would not be overjoyed with the enhanced self-confidence, intensified awareness, and increased ability to tolerate pain that comes with taking anabolic steroids. The problem is, when

Table 4.3 Physiological Effects of Using Anabolic Steroids

Anabolic changes attributed to anabolic steroids

- Increased skeletal muscle mass
- Increased organ mass
- Increased hemoglobin concentration
- Increased red blood cell mass
- Control of the distribution of body fat
- Increased calcium in the bones
- Increased total body nitrogen retention
- Increased electrolyte retention
- Increased protein synthesis

Androgenic changes attributed to anabolic steroids

- Increased density and pattern of body hair
- Increased density and distribution of facial hair
- Deepening voice
- Increased oil production of the sebaceous glands
- Increased sexual desire
- Fluid retention
- Hypertension
- Non-scarring acne
- Cystic acne
- Oily skin
- Facial pore enlargement
- Scalp hair loss
- Decreased breast size (women)
- Breast development (men)
- Menstrual irregularities (women)
- Clitoral enlargement (women)
- Testicular atrophy (men)

Adapted from Taylor 1985.[2]

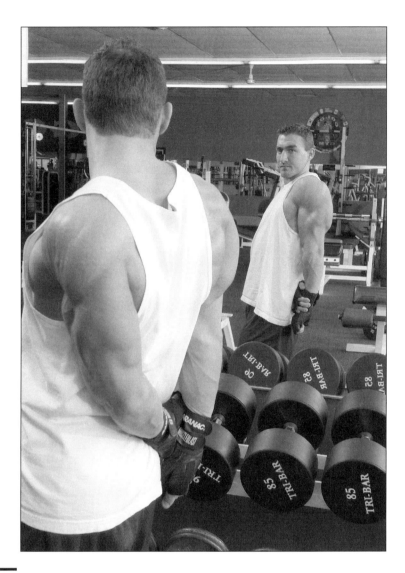

You will never feel better about your body than when you build muscle tissue the natural way.

these positive psychological changes are eventually overridden by negative changes, the situation can create an adverse and incredibly volatile situation. Violent and erratic mood swings and intolerance of others can ignite hostility and aggression, which ultimately lead to a path of destruction.

Another problem is that the positive psychological benefits of taking anabolic steroids can be addictive. If taking a drug could make you more self-confident and renew your passion to train, would you do it? Like the physical benefits of taking anabolic steroids, the psychological benefits are difficult to give up. The "downer" of cycling off the drugs is simply too difficult for most bodybuilders to handle. Instead, they keep using them in larger and larger dosages to maintain a positive psychological outlook. Table 4.4 lists the psychological changes that occur in bodybuilders who use and then cease using anabolic steroids.

Psychological Benefits Without the Use of Drugs

So far, I have advocated the importance of a healthy, muscle-building diet, a scientifically based training program, adequate rest and sleep, and a positive mind-set if you want to reach the peak of body development. Even if you do all of these things, however, you will still not be able to match the anabolic benefits of taking steroids. Simply put: anabolic steroids are extremely effective in making the necessary physiological changes for advanced muscular size and strength.

Psychological benefits, however, are another story. The human mind is powerful. Of the positive psychological changes that accompany anabolic steroid use—increased aggressiveness, mental intensity, energy level, tolerance of pain, focus, desire to train, self-esteem, and ability to train with greater intensity—there is not one that cannot be developed through a systematic mental-training program. You can learn to focus your attention to minimize distraction. You can use your mind to overcome the excruciating pain that comes with intense workouts. You can use the power of self-coaching to improve your self-esteem.

Yes, anabolic steroids can have a positive effect on your mind and your personality, but these effects usually go too far. Increased hostility toward others, not to mention violent mood swings and outbursts, can irreversibly damage your relationships with friends and loved ones. Why take the chance of ruining your life when you do not have to? You can have that same positive outlook on life and bodybuilding without the financial cost or risks of steroid use. Trust me, you will never feel better about yourself for the way you look than when you build your body the natural way.

Because the high dosages of steroids typically taken by bodybuilders have such serious side effects, it is imperative that bodybuilders seriously evaluate whether the benefits outweigh the risks before considering an anabolic steroid program. Although some effects are temporary and reversible, many are permanent. Bodybuilders must ask themselves whether they are prepared to live with those effects for the rest of their lives.

Your body is a finely tuned machine and like any machine it needs fuel to keep running. A clear understanding of which fuel to give your body can become blurred by the constant barrage of nutritional messages pumped out in the media. The better you are at sifting through the piles of useless and inaccurate nutritional information the better off you will be. Once you have established an optimal eating pattern for muscle growth, then the mental skills that you will discover in the rest of this book will be that much more beneficial and rewarding.

Table 4.4 Potential Psychological Alterations Induced in Men Taking Anabolic Steroids

Alterations while on steroids

- Increased sex drive
- Increased aggressiveness
- Increased appetite
- Increased tendency for hostility
- Increased mental intensity
- Increased energy level
- Increased tolerance of pain
- Increased tendency toward "one-track" thinking
- Increased desire to train
- Increased tendency toward uncontrolled temperment
- Increased self-esteem
- Increased ability to train with greater intensity
- Increased inability to accept failure or poor athletic performance
- Decreased inhibitions toward further drug use
- Sleeping disturbances and nightmares
- Psychological dependency on anabolic steroids

Alterations after cessation of steroids

- Decreased sex drive
- Decreased appetite
- Chemical depression
- Decreased self-esteem
- Decreased desire to train
- Increased desire to take the drugs again
- Slowly improved ability to control behavior
- Decreased aggressiveness
- Slow return to normal sleeping patterns
- Energy levels slowly returning to normal
- Decreased mental intensity
- Increased tendency toward apathy
- Decreased ability to train with intensity

Adapted from Taylor 1985.[3]

CHAPTER 5

Warming Up and Tuning In to the Body

Most coaches and athletes recognize the need to warm up. Even the most casual fitness buffs make a show of jogging a few paces and touching their toes before joining their training partners. They know, at least in theory, that stretching and warming up muscles reduces the risk of injury. Because bodybuilding places incredible demands on both the body and the psyche, bodybuilders need to warm up physically as well as psychologically. This chapter examines the physiological and psychological rationale for an appropriate warm-up and outlines things to consider when designing a warm-up, including the pre-workout routine as well as mind-body interplay during various warm-up techniques.

Physiological Demands of Bodybuilding

It is clear to anyone who engages in a serious strength-training program that the physiological demands of bodybuilding are great. The mission of bodybuilders is packing on hard muscle without increasing body fat. For muscles to grow, there must be an enlargement of muscle fibers. This increase in muscle fiber, called hypertrophy, increases the ability to develop force and execute heavy lifts. Hypertrophy is influenced by the amount of time in training. That is, strength increases during early stages of training do not necessarily lead to hypertrophy. It is only after one to two months of training that increases in muscle fiber begin to match increases in strength.

Hypertrophy is also influenced by training intensity. Experienced body-builders achieve increases in hypertrophy only when training intensity is optimized. Indeed, for experienced bodybuilders, increases in muscle strength are easier to achieve than increases in muscle mass. What does this mean for the serious bodybuilder? If it means that if you want to increase muscle strength and size, you must train at maximum intensity most of the time.

At a basic level, bodybuilding is about optimally stressing your bones, muscles, and connective tissue with weight training and then allowing your body adequate time for recuperation and renewal. This will produce both an increase in muscular size and overall strength.

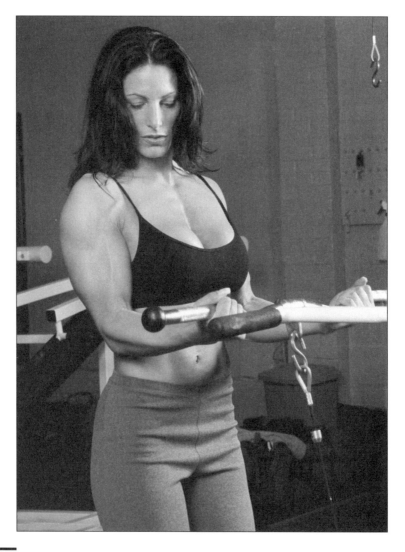

For maximum growth to occur you must place your muscles, bones, and connective tissue under stress.

You have probably heard that to reduce the effects of osteoporosis, a degenerative bone disease, it is best to engage in weight-bearing exercise. Your bones are rigid, but they are also active and have the capacity for growth and regeneration if damaged. The more a bone is stressed with the compressive forces of weight-bearing exercise, the greater the increase in bone mass. Larger muscle mass also contributes to increased bone mass by forcing the bone to provide sufficient support for the enlarged muscles. In sum, any increase or decrease in muscle strength or mass will result in a corresponding decrease or increase in bone mass.

Weights used in bodybuilding training programs are lighter than those used in strength-training or powerlifting programs, but they are heavy enough to elicit concentric or eccentric contraction failure. An eccentric contraction occurs when force is applied against a lengthening muscle. For example, a bodybuilder who slowly lowers the weight in a bicep curl is executing an eccentric contraction. A concentric contraction is the opposite of the eccentric contraction and occurs when the muscle is shortening, such as when the bodybuilder raises the weight in a bicep curl. Lighter weights used in a bodybuilding training program allows the bodybuilder to perform more reps (6 to 12) than would be typical in a strength-training program (3 to 5 reps). Bodybuilders also take shorter rests between sets. It is not unusual for a bodybuilder to perform as many as 20 successive sets that focus on one muscle group. High-volume training with shorter rest periods seems to be optimal for hypertrophy.

The hypertrophy process, as described by William J. Kraemer in *Essentials of Strength Training and Conditioning,* is the following: "Hypertrophy involves an increase in the synthesis of the contractile proteins actin and myosin within the myofibril as well as an increase in the number of myofibrils within a muscle fiber. The new myofilaments are added to the external layers of the myofibril, resulting in an increase in its diameter."[1] Basically, bodybuilding breaks down muscle fibers and rebuilds them. That is why training must be intense enough to break down muscle fibers and the rest periods must be long enough to allow for the rebuilding process.

The primary stimuli for connective tissue growth are the mechanical forces created during physical activity. Stronger muscles pull harder on the bony attachments, increasing the strength and size of the connective tissue. So, as with bone and muscle, the training must be intense enough to stimulate connective tissue growth. According to *Essentials of Strength Training and Conditioning,* research indicates that weight training increases collagen fibril diameter, increases the number of covalent cross-links within a fiber of increased diameter, increases the number of collagen fibrils, and heightens the collagen fibril-packing density. It seems that as a response to body building, connective tissue adapts, allowing it to withstand greater tensional force.[2]

Psychological Demands of Bodybuilding

When I was coaching competitive swimming, I always thought it was strange that younger athletes were nervous about swimming distance events (200 meters and longer). They would want to compete in sprint events because they considered them easier. Their frame of mind was that shorter was better because they would only have to work hard for a minute or less. No matter what I did, I could not convince them that distance races were in fact easier because they allowed for different strategies and mistake correction during the race.

What these young athletes could not seem to grasp was that being a good sprinter in swimming, running, or cycling requires an extremely high level of training intensity. In many ways, anaerobic (sprint) training is very difficult, placing high physiological and psychological demands on the athlete. Bodybuilding is just such an anaerobic activity in which individual sets may last up to 90 seconds. Sure, it is possible to "go through the motions" during a set and not experience the type of physical discomfort or pain associated with muscle growth. This is true of any type of exercise and is fine if you want a body that looks like it "just went through the motions." If you want a hard-packed, ripped physique, however, you will have to learn to work at a high intensity level during those anaerobic sets. Shorter is not easier, but it is different.

The difference between aerobic training and anaerobic training can be compared to the difference between short and long labor periods in the birthing process. You have probably heard of women who have had to endure 36 hours of labor when delivering a new baby. Is it possible that they experienced the same level of pain and discomfort as those who had only a few hours of labor? Based on the experience of my wife, other women I have spoken with, and extensive research in the study of pain, the answer is no. It is obviously painful for women to give birth, but the way they experience pain is unique. Women who have short labor experience an intense pain for only a short time. Women who have long labor experience a dull ache that intensifies as the moment of birth approaches. The experience of pain in labor is unique to each woman and there is no doubt that different levels of pain intensity will be experienced. It is also true that the time between contractions will vary in length and intensity. Most women find that the time between contractions is just the calm before the storm as they physically and mentally prepare for the next contraction. No one type of labor is "better," certainly; they are just different.

While certainly not as intense, bodybuilding can be likened to the pain experienced during short labor: pain can be very intense but will immediately go away after each set. If you want to increase the size of your muscular frame, you will have to be mentally prepared for intense, physical discomfort. But rest assured, it will go away as soon as the set is complete.

I have now written at length about the psychological demands placed on a bodybuilder during an individual set, but what about the rest of the workout, day, and week? Bodybuilding is a lifestyle of commitment and strong desire to improve the way you look and feel. That means bodybuilders need to remain focused during workouts and be able to stay disciplined in their nutritional habits and training patterns. Bodybuilding is a difficult road to follow—in fact, most will choose an easier path—but for those who have the mental fortitude and desire to build their bodies, the rewards are plentiful.

Mental Preparation for Training

To develop to your potential, you must be mentally and emotionally prepared. It is a good idea to begin your mental preparation hours before a training session, and days before a competition. The problem is that most bodybuilders have no idea what to do. Too often, bodybuilders arrive at the gym after a hard day at work with little thought about the purpose of the workout. Their focus is on anything but muscular development, which means they are unprepared to get the most out of their workouts. Many bodybuilders spend countless hours in the gym because they have failed to prepare. They try to overcome their lack of preparation by putting in more time, which is simply wasting time.

To perform your best in training or in competition, it is essential that you prepare well. The development of a pre-workout routine is essential to optimal bodybuilding, because it allows you to redirect your attention from outside distractions to those factors that play a key role in your muscular development. Such a pre-workout routine must include self-awareness activities and the opportunity for mental preparation. An example of a pre-workout routine is shown in table 5.1.

The main purpose of a pre-workout routine is achieving peak performance, that is, executing more sets and reps and lifting heavier weights. Peak performance is a function of both physical and mental factors. For peak performance to occur, it is essential that you master weight-lifting techniques, including physical conditioning. As indicated in chapter 1, however, few bodybuilders achieve optimal muscular development.

For peak muscular development, the mind must be developed and trained to interact with the body. Most personal trainers and bodybuilders agree that the mind accounts for at least 40 percent of success in bodybuilding, although many believe it accounts for even more. The more muscular the frame, the more significant the role that mental skills play in further development. This is because bodybuilders who have achieved some success are that much closer to realizing their potential. Thus, further developments require high levels of mental fortitude and toughness.

In elite bodybuilding competitions, it is usually the person who is strongest mentally, leading up to the competition, who will be declared the victor.

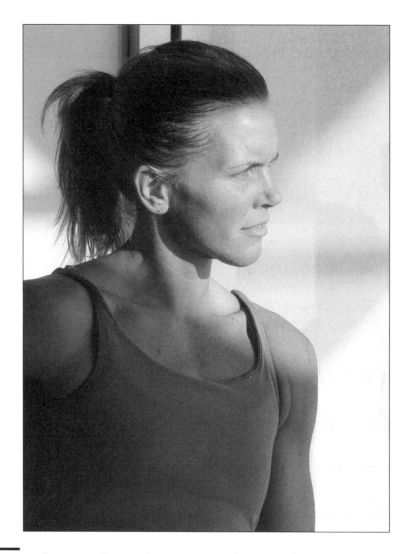

Being mentally prepared goes a long way toward ensuring bodybuilding success.

Studies conducted with Olympic athletes have consistently shown that when physical, technical, and mental preparation were assessed, only mental preparation played a significant role in their success. By making sure that you are mentally prepared to train and compete, you also ensure that the muscular size and definition you have worked so hard to develop will be exhibited most effectively in shows and competitions, or even at the beach.

The book *Peak Performance: Mental Training Techniques of the World's Greatest Athletes*, outlines a study of hundreds of elite athletes, identifying eight mental and physical conditions characteristic of the way athletes feel when they are doing something extraordinarily well. The following is a list of mental and physical conditions.

Table 5.1   Pre-Workout Routine

Activity	Time	Purpose
1. Travel to gym	10-20 min.	Reflect on internal distractions. Determine goals for workout. Mentally prepare and self-motivate for intense workout.
2. Arrive at gym	5-7 min.	Discover and deal with external distractions. Deal with distractions prior to workout. Arrive at least 10 minutes before workout. Discuss distractions with training partner.
3. Light cardiovascular warm-up	5-7 min.	Prepare body for physical effort. Attune body with the mind. Review goals for the workout.
4. Stretching	4-6 min.	Prepare specific muscle groups for training. Focus attention on next 45 minutes of intense muscle-building exercise.
5. Light warm-up sets	2-4 min.	Go through motions of specific exercises. Narrow focus to specific muscle groups and exercises.

6. You are now ready for an intense, body-sculpting workout!

1. Mental relaxation is described as a sense of inner calm. Some athletes also reported the sensation of time slowing down and having a high degree of concentration. By contrast, athletes who said that everything was happening too fast reported a loss of concentration and a sense of being out of control.

2. Physical relaxation can be described as muscles feeling loose and movement feeling fluid and sure.

3. Confidence and optimism are characterized by having a positive attitude and feelings of self-confidence. Athletes who reported this condition were able to remain poised and maintain feelings of strength and control, even during potentially threatening challenges.

4. Possessing a focus on the present can be described as a sense of harmony stemming from the body and mind working as one. These athletes reported no thoughts of the past or future and a sense of their bodies performing automatically, without conscious or deliberate effort.

5. High energy is described as a highly energized state with feelings of joy, ecstasy, intensity, and being "charged" or "hot."

6. Hyperawareness is described as being acutely aware of both the body and the surrounding environment. Some athletes also reported an uncanny ability to know what other athletes were going to do, and thus an ability to respond accordingly.

7. Automatic control, described as being "in the zone," exists when the body and mind are automatically executing every move correctly, without conscious control of the action.

8. Detachment is described as being "in the cocoon," a feeling of being completely detached from the external environment and any potential distractions. Athletes who reported this condition also said that they felt a sense of having complete access to all their powers and skills, including focus, power, and control.

Developing Your Own Pre-Workout Routine

A pre-workout routine will help you prepare for and deal with the critical factors that can affect your workouts. To ensure effective mental and emotional control before and during a training session, it is important to be able to keep these factors in check. Critical factors include your gym, equipment, training partner, the purpose of the workout, and mental readiness.

Your Gym

The gym environment can be distracting, neutral, or helpful. The gym may be too old, too cold, too warm, too small, or too glossy with lots of mirrors, chrome, and bright colors. It may have loud air fans, archaic equipment, inadequate air circulation, or too many mirrors. It is easy to find an annoyance or distraction in any gym. But rather than look for things that can negatively affect your workouts, why not learn to use your gym's idiosyncrasies to your advantage? The better you become at training in "less than ideal" conditions, the greater your ability to sculpt your body in any environment you might find yourself in.

Within the gym, of course, other people may be the biggest distraction or annoyance. Constantly comparing yourself with other bodybuilders or checking out the "hot" body at the shoulder press will only distract you from reaching your goals. Give yourself a few minutes at the start of every training session to look around the gym, notice what is different, and check out fellow bodybuilders. Afterward, you will be able to focus on what is important: training intensity.

Equipment

In bodybuilding, as in most sports, equipment is crucial for success. If the equipment is not properly adjusted and in good working order, it is difficult to perform at your best. If you find faulty equipment in your gym, speak to the gym owner or manager. In addition, make sure you take care of your own equipment; your gloves, lifting belt, shoes, and clothing. Anything that is loose, broken, or worn down may distract you. Worse, it might lead to an accident or injury.

In addition to ensuring its proper operation, it is also important to calibrate your equipment. Look over the equipment you plan to use during your workout. Do you need to make any adjustments? Can you set up the equipment (correct amount of weight, pins in the right places, right seat angles) before you begin your workout? It is extremely distracting when equipment does not work right or feels uncomfortable during a workout.

Training Partner

As much as you are able, you will need to focus on task-related information while preparing for your workout. Your training partner, however, may arrive at the gym wanting to talk about the events of the past few days or week. Allow yourself some time to talk in a free, unrestricted manner. Then gently direct your conversation to task-related topics. A few minutes is all that should be devoted to discussing school, weekend parties, friends, or work. After that, all conversation should be centered on your workout and the goals you would both like to accomplish.

This is the time to come together as a synchronized unit of strength and conditioning. A partnership that is well attuned to the other's bodybuilding needs will accomplish much more than any one individual can. (See chapter 8 for more about getting the most out of your experience with a training partner.)

The Purpose of the Workout

You may have already begun to think about your short-term and long-term goals for this year, but have you thought about setting goals for each and every workout? You must know the purpose of each workout and how it fits

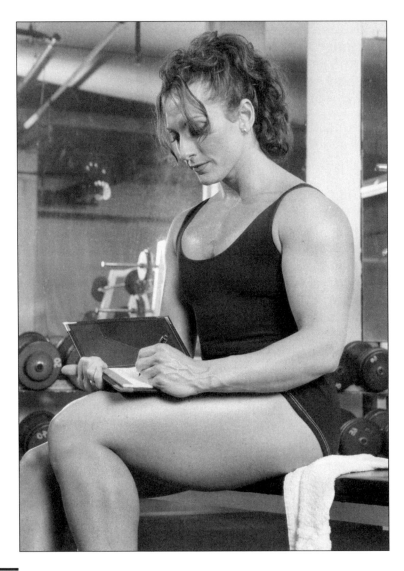

A logbook can be particularly helpful in keeping your workouts focused.

into your overall plan for muscular development. You may find that using a training log, which you complete before each workout, will be extremely helpful in staying focused. Such a log can also be helpful in your mental preparation and could include information such as the purpose of the workout, the number of sets and reps you intend to complete, the type of exercises, the planned rest periods, and the types of food you will ingest before, during, and after the workout. Once you have recorded these things in your log, stick with your plans and work them as hard as you can.

Note, however, that using a log does not mean that you should never change your plans or that you should not be innovative in your program.

What it does mean is that any changes in your training program should be made in the quiet of your home or office, not during the middle of your workout.

Mental Readiness

The final component in any effective pre-workout routine is mental preparation. Every bodybuilder is different, so each person must mentally prepare in whatever manner will ensure his or her optimal mental readiness. Through personal experience and interactions with other bodybuilders, you have probably learned what you need to achieve readiness. Some bodybuilders become highly anxious before a workout and simply need to relax. Others are already too laid-back and need to energize themselves. Some bodybuilders rely heavily on visualization, stretching, and massage, while others need loud, uplifting music to invigorate them. Whatever the mental preparation, identify the techniques that best prepare you for an effective workout.

Be aware that even though you may be comfortable with the way you prepare for a workout, you may not be employing the best method. For example, listening to loud music may energize you, but it may not help you to be mentally prepared. Loud music can cause you to be overaroused and distract you from critical cues while lifting. If you want to try a different mental-preparation technique, try it out before a noncritical training session. If it turns out that this new technique is effective, then you can use it before a critical workout or competition.

Developing a pre-training routine is a personal process. Through trial and error, you will discover what suits you best. An effective pre-workout routine typically consists of minimizing distractions, focusing, and dealing with any factors that may adversely affect your performance. Some of these, such as faulty equipment or too much physical tension, can be addressed during the pre-training routine. Others, such as loud music or other people in the gym, are out of your control. These factors you must deal with by changing your response to them during your pre-workout routine. Note: Changing your response to outside factors may actually help your performance. For example, as you turn your attention from external distractions to internal thoughts and feelings, and then back to your training partner and goals, you are improving your focus and concentration.

Mind/Body Interplay During Physical Warm-Up

It is not only possible to connect the mind and body during your physical warm-up; it is also imperative for bodybuilding success. Mind-body harmony is best accomplished by performing your regular physical warm-up routine at the same time as you prepare mentally. This is an important part of the pre-workout routine. This section explains the use of kinaesthetic imagery during warm-up and gives you some examples of the mind-body interplay.

Have you ever woken up in the middle of a dream and not knowing whether the dream was real? Have you ever noticed that your heart and breathing rates increase while you watch a scary movie? These experiences, called "kinaesthetic" experiences, affect the entire body. The reason dreams can seem so real is that the body responds to a dream in the same way that it would to a real-life event. If someone were chasing you in a dream your heart would beat faster, as though you were actually running.

Kinaesthetic imagery is a form of imagery that requires you to feel yourself perform. Whatever you do in your "mind's eye" is mirrored in the physical world. Kinaesthetic imagery excites the same neurological pathways that actual performance does. This does not mean that you can imagine beyond your physical ability and it will happen, of course. Imagery rehearsal will only enable you to do what you are already physically capable of doing. But remember the role of mental skills outlined in chapter 1: to get you as close to your bodybuilding potential as possible. Imagery rehearsal is one of those skills.

A type of kinaesthetic imagery involves the use of a metaphorical image. Bodybuilders about to execute the squat may envision themselves as a powerful bull pulling a heavy boulder, or you might see yourself as a smooth-flowing river as you move from one pose to another during a contest. The number of metaphors is limited only by your imagination.

The physical warm-up is a perfect time to conjure an image you want to use in your workout. Imagining that you are a gladiator preparing for an upcoming contest may help you to lift with renewed intensity. To get the most from metaphorical imagery, be sure that the images you use are in line with your training goals and personality.

Kinaesthetic imagery can be used while stretching or stationary cycling, during the first few "light" sets of a workout, while relaxing and listening to music, even when sitting in a hot tub. In fact, it is almost impossible to find an activity or place where kinaesthetic imagery cannot be effective.

To begin using kinaesthetic imagery, close your eyes and begin to see yourself performing an exercise or posing routine. Feel the body sensations as you execute each movement in your mind. Feel the bar in your hands, the motion of every muscle, your breathing, your heart rate, the sweat running down your face, and the resistance of the weight. Feel yourself power through the set and notice how your muscles begin to tire as you push through each rep. Feel yourself applying more and more force against the bar as you complete the final rep. Notice how your muscles burn as you finish the set. Finally, feel how your "jellied" muscles respond after the bar has been placed back on the rack. At first you may find it difficult to "feel" the physical sensations of the exercise, but the imagery will become more vivid and effective as you practice. For further discussion on the role of imagery in bodybuilding success, see chapter 10.

Warm Up for Success: Beth Horn

Beth Horn is an IFBB fitness professional and personal trainer. Her pictures have appeared in many fitness and bodybuilding magazines, including *Muscle & Fitness, Ironman,* and *Oxygen.* Beth is the overall National Fitness Champion (NFC) for 2000 and can be seen on her website (**http://www.bethhorn.com**). She offers these comments about an effective warm-up:

It is important to warm up the muscles before weight training to get the blood flowing. When I work with clients, I have them do a five-minute warm-up on an aerobic machine, such as the elliptical trainer or stair climber. More often than not, they comment on how much better they feel when they increase their heart rate and get the blood flowing through the muscles. Even if they are planning to focus their workout on cardiovascular development, it is best to warm up the muscles three to five minutes and slowly increase the heart rate before taking it to the next level.

Once the light cardiovascular activity is done, a good warm-up for the working muscles is a very light set with the muscles you are about to train. For example, when I am going to train my upper body, I like to start with 15 shoulder presses using a light weight. Bench pressing with light weight (20 to 30 percent of your max) is also a good upper body warm-up. For the lower body, I find that squats are an excellent warm-up. Doing squats (15 to 20 reps) with little or no weight should warm up your legs and get you ready for more intense training. If the workout is going to be a heavy one, you may want to do several warm-up sets to be safe and really get the muscles warm. Using the bench press as an example again, you may want to add 5 to 10 pounds for each warm-up set. You may need 3 to 5 sets to build up to the heavier weights.

I also like to stretch slightly to warm up before certain activities. Before I dance, do gymnastics, or perform a cardiovascular activity, for example, I like to stretch out my hamstrings, quads, and calves before getting into the routine.

If you want to get the most out of your lifting, it is important to focus mentally before your weight training. I focus on the muscles I am working, as well as the results I am striving for. I also concentrate on the outcome and think about upcoming fitness competitions. It is always helpful to write your goals down, as well as keep them in the forefront of your mind. I believe that you can do anything you put your mind to, and that includes what you want your body to look like. If you can see that body, you can achieve it!

Light Cardiovascular Exercise

Go into any fitness center in the world and you will see people riding a stationary bike, running on a treadmill, and using the stair stepper and elliptical trainer. Many use this equipment for aerobic conditioning and burning body fat. Bodybuilders, however, use it as part of their physical warm-up.

A light cardiovascular warm-up can be much more than simply spinning the pedals or jogging on a treadmill. Light cardiovascular exercise combined with the right mind-set can become a powerful tool to prepare for the intensity required in any muscle-building workout. Table 5.2 illustrates the mind-body interplay during a 10-minute cycling warm-up. While specifically detailing the movements of cycling, this example is intended to show the intricate mind-body relationship during any routine warm-up activity and to guide you in creating your own powerful, mind-body warm-up.

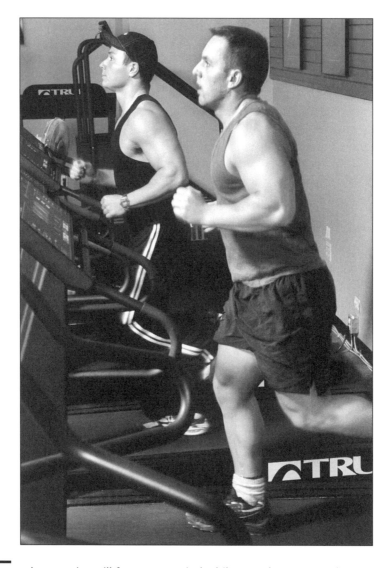

Cardiovascular exercise will focus your mind while you plan your workout.

| | **Table 5.2** | **Mind–Body Interplay During Stationary Cycling** | |

Table 5.2   Mind–Body Interplay During Stationary Cycling

Time	Cycling action	Mind response
2 min.	Easy spinning of the pedals, nice relaxed grip on the handlebars. Heart rate should be about 120 bpm.	• Determine your goals for the upcoming workout. • Survey the gym and focus on the equipment you will need to accomplish your goals. • Determine the length of workout and intensity level necessary for goal achievement.
3 min.	Pedal tension is increased. Breathing rate increases and the body begins to perspire. Heart rate should be approximately 140-150 bpm.	• Conduct a quick body scan (see chapter 10) to help you develop kinaesthetic awareness of your body. • Close your eyes and use the colored body parts exercise (see chapter 10) to help you mentally isolate the muscle groups you will focus on during the workout.
3 min.	Pedal tension is increased once again and sprint/easy spin alternations begin. 20 seconds of sprinting (90% effort) with 20 seconds of easy spinning. Heart rate should be approximately 160-175 bpm.	• Open your eyes. Begin to imagine that each sprint is a set of weights and the easy spinning is the rest period between sets. • As you sprint kinaesthetically, "feel" yourself executing every rep with intense passion.

(continued)

Table 5.2	(continued)	

Time	Cycling action	Mind response
1 min.	Pedal tension is decreased. Breathing and heart rates begin to normalize. Heart rate should be approximately 140 bpm.	• Visualize the image that you want to portray. Is it a powerful bull, or a pump filling your muscles with blood? • Feel and see that image in your mind's eye. You are a powerful bull, ready to push hard against the weights.
1 min.	Pedal tension is further decreased. Easy spinning as heart and breathing rates normalize. Heart rate should fall below 120 before getting off the bike.	• Slowly come out of your visualization and once again begin to concentrate on the gym. • Looking around the gym, you are now physically warm and mentally ready to begin the mass building process.

Stretching

The goal of stretching is to physically prepare the body for exercise and prevent possible injury. After a workout, stretching takes on the additional role of enhancing flexibility. Proper stretching lengthens muscle tissue, making it less "tight" and therefore less prone to trauma and tears. Here are a few tips to get the most benefit from stretching.

• Do some light cardiovascular exercise before stretching. A warm muscle is much more easily stretched than a cold muscle. Always warm up first to get some blood circulating and into the muscles. Cardiovascular activity should be slow and rhythmic, such as slow cycling or walking, and should be done for at least five minutes so that the body has sufficient time to elevate the temperature of the muscles.

• Use static stretching. There are many different types of stretches that can be done on your own or with a partner, including static, dynamic, ballistic, and proprioceptive neuromuscular facilitation (PNF). PNF is a form of stretching that is partner assisted. Each type of stretching serves a purpose, whether it be preparation for training or flexibility enhancement, but the most appropriate type for a bodybuilding warm-up is probably static stretching. Static stretching involves a slow, gradual, and controlled elongation of the muscle though the full range of motion. Stretch until you can stretch no further without pain, hold the stretch for 15 to 30 seconds, then rest 15 seconds and repeat 2 or 3 times.

Most research shows that stretching before each workout is most beneficial. Frequent stretching will help you to avoid the muscular imbalances, cramps, tightness, and soreness that can accompany the bodybuilding lifestyle.

• Stretch between weightlifting sets. Experienced bodybuilders know that rest and muscle recovery are crucial for muscle growth. Why not use the time between sets for something better than talking to the good-looking person at the leg press? Frank Zane, a two-time Mr. Olympia winner, does just that. He uses the rest time between sets to enhance muscle recovery and increase flexibility.

Most bodybuilders will tell you that a stretching routine feels good and can be a very relaxing part of the workout, but few understand that stretching does more than just feel good. Stretching, when combined with a proper mind-set, can set you up for the best workouts you have ever had. Check out table 5.3 to see how a standard leg-stretching routine can be enhanced with the power of the mind. Again, this example can be adapted to any stretching routine. By taking advantage of the mind-body relationship, using it to suit your goals, personality, and environment, you will go a long way to reaching peak performance during your workouts.

Warm-Up Sets

If you are not in the habit of using the first few sets of every workout to further warm your muscles, you need to be. Article after article in muscle magazines will tell you that the first few sets of every workout are critical to promote the neuromuscular adaptation necessary for more intense muscle-building exercise. The warm-up sets (the first two sets of each training session and the first set of each subsequent exercise) should be done using a weight that is 30 to 50 percent of your one-rep maximum. It is also a great time to connect your mind and body by visualizing the exercise at the same time you perform it.

As you move toward each exercise station, begin to imagine what it is going to feel like when you move the weight. Even though the weight is "light" and easy to move, feel every muscle coming together as a synchronized force. Remember to use your nonvisual senses to experience how it feels and what you hear. Close your eyes as you lift and then open and close your eyes several times until you begin to get a kinaesthetic awareness of the

Table 5.3 Mind-Body Interplay During Leg Stretching

Stretch	Execution	Mind response
Supine knee flex	Lie on your back on a table with your leg and hip as near the edge as possible. Pull your other thigh and knee firmly toward your chest until your lower back flattens against the table. Let your other leg hang in a relaxed position over the edge. Switch legs.	• Determine your goals for the upcoming workout. • Survey the gym and focus on the equipment you will need to accomplish your goals. • Determine the length of workout and the intensity level necessary for goal achievement.
Hip adductor stretch	Lie on your back on a firm surface with your hips and knees bent and feet flat. Gently let your knees fall apart, keeping the soles of your feet together until you feel an inner thigh stretch.	• Conduct a quick body scan (see chapter 10) to help you develop kinesthetic awareness of your body.
Hamstring stretch	Lie in a doorway, keeping your back straight and flat against the floor. Raise one leg against the wall until you feel a gentle stretch behind the knee. Keep the leg on the floor straight, aligned with your back. Switch legs.	• Run through the Black Box Visualization (see chapter 10) to eliminate distractions that will affect the workout. • Use this time to clear your mind and begin to focus on the next 45 minutes in the gym.

Stretch	Execution	Mind response
Semi-straddle stretch	Sit with your upper body vertical and your legs straight. Place the sole of your left foot on the inside of the right knee, resting the left knee on the floor. Lean forward from the waist and grasp your right toes with your right hand, slightly pulling the toes toward the upper body. Release your toes and relax your foot. Lean forward again, this time grasping your right ankle, and pull your chest toward the right leg. Hold for 15 seconds. Switch legs and repeat the pattern.	• Using the body awareness technique (see chapter 10), begin to see and feel yourself lifting weight with power and fluidity.
Side quadriceps stretch	Lie on your left side with both legs straight and your left arm on the floor by your head. Flex your right leg, with the heel of the right foot moving toward your buttocks. Grasp the front of the ankle with your right hand and pull your foot toward the buttocks. Stop if you experience pain in the right knee. Move the knee backward and slightly upward until the stretch is felt. Hold for 15 seconds. Repeat on the other side.	• Begin to visualize yourself going through the workout with a renewed intensity and passion. • Use positive visualization (see chapter 10) to self-confirm your power, strength, and symmetry. You are a great body-builder, and you must continue to tell yourself that while you are getting ready to work out.
Forward lunge stretch	Standing, take a long step forward with your right leg and flex the right knee until it is directly over the right foot. Keep the right foot flat on the floor and the back leg straight. Keep the torso upright and rest your hands on your hips or front leg. Slowly lower the hips down and forward. Hold for 15 seconds. Repeat with the left leg.	• Visualize the image that you want to portray. Is it a ferocious lion, or a pump filling your muscles with blood? • Begin to see and feel that image. Believe that you are that lion about to attack the weights with a vengeance.

(continued)

Table 5.3	(continued)	
Stretch	**Execution**	**Mind response**
Calf stretch	Stand at arm's length from a wall with your palms flat against the wall. Slowly bend your elbows and lean toward the wall. Keep your legs with knees straight with the heels flat on the floor. Hold for 15 seconds.	• Slowly come out of your visualization and once again begin to concentrate on the gym. • Looking around the gym, you are now physically warm and mentally ready to begin the mass building process.

skill. This experience will switch you from imagery to reality several times over a short period of time. Now you are ready to begin your "real" sets with an aggressive fervor.

It would be easy to simply go through the motions during a workout and walk away believing you had pushed yourself to the limit and had forced your muscles to grow. The truth is, if you do not take the workout seriously, you are wasting your time. Many bodybuilders go through their workouts without direction or focus, and many of them never seem to get any bigger, stronger, or more defined. By learning to synthesize your mind and body during the warm-up, however, you will be able train with renewed intensity, which will produce that bulk, definition, and symmetry you desire. This mind-body interplay during warm-up is an essential part of coaching yourself, the topic of the next chapter.

CHAPTER 6

Working Out, Training Within

Imagination is invaluable when it comes to the development of athletic skills and strategies. Indeed, it can mean the difference between a successful performance and a bad performance. If you cannot imagine yourself performing a skill or achieving success, you will literally be unable to do it. Have you ever woken up in a sweat after a nightmare or had butterflies just thinking about that speech you had to give the next day? The body reacts in a similar way to things imagined as it does to real events. The subconscious is not capable of distinguishing between real success and imagined success.

It has been said that if you believe you can do something, you can. Likewise, if you believe you cannot do something, you will not be able to. No matter what you believe, negative or positive, it will become a self-fulfilling prophecy and control your future behavior. As a bodybuilder, if you believe that you will never be able to increase the size of your arms or decrease your body fat, you are probably right.

This chapter is about learning to coach yourself through individual workouts and, in general, the bodybuilding lifestyle. You will learn about the role of negative and positive self-talk in achieving your goals, along with how to use self-talk to your advantage. You will also learn to develop a self-coaching plan.

Using Positive Self-Talk

Self-talk is not limited to positive thinking alone. In fact, self-talk can be used in many other ways to help you become a better bodybuilder. You can use self-talk to learn new lifting techniques, correct bad habits, prepare for a performance, focus your attention, improve your mood, confuse your muscles, and build competence and self-confidence.

Self-Talk for New Lifting Techniques

In the initial stages of learning a new technique, positive self-talk about certain key aspects of the skill can significantly improve your skill acquisition. For example, when learning eccentric bicep contractions, you will need to remind yourself to lower the weight very slowly (five to eight seconds), to stay controlled, to move slowly through the entire range of motion, and to remain focused on the biceps throughout each full rep.

As you begin to master the technique, self-talk should move from a focus on lifting mechanics to mental fortitude and positive thinking. Failure to make the transition from mechanical self-talk to focused self-talk can cause "paralysis by analysis." Most common with novice bodybuilders and those learning new techniques, "paralysis by analysis" occurs when bodybuilders fail to get the most out of a rep or set because they are too focused on the mechanical aspects of a lifting technique.

Self-Talk for Changing Bad Habits

As an experienced bodybuilder, you likely have ingrained bad habits that affect your training. Bad habits could include reinforcing a negative self-image, wasting time in the gym, and "cheating" on exercises. These bad habits may be difficult to change, but it is imperative that you change them if you want optimal muscular development. Like changing negative attitudes, changing bad habits involves unlearning automatic responses that are no longer effective and replacing them with new responses. In addition to conscious control, this requires self-talk. For example, if you find yourself getting into a full-blown conversation with another bodybuilder at the gym, use self-talk to steer yourself toward the desired outcome (time-effective training) and away from the undesirable behavior (wasting time talking to others).

It is like trying to avoid hitting another car while driving. If you focus on the car ahead, you will probably drive right into it. If you focus your eyes on the open space ahead of and beside the car, however, you will likely steer your vehicle past the car and into the open space. The same thing can happen in the gym. For example, rather than visualize yourself hammering out the reps (what you *do* want to do), you think about not completing the set (what you do *not* want to do). Focusing on what you desire keeps negative thoughts and images at bay, and makes it easier for you to achieve what you want.

Self-Talk for Focus

It is easy to be distracted in fitness centers and bodybuilding gyms. Music, chatter, mirrors, television, and the plethora of fit, toned bodies can make it

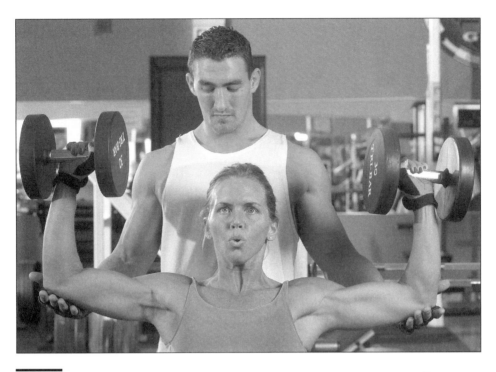

Learn to filter out all the distractions in the gym and focus on your workout. This allows you to maintain intensity.

challenging to stay on track. By using a specific set of attentional cues—breathing patterns, the "pump" in your muscles, and encouragement from others—you can return your focus to the thing that is most important: your workout.

Learn to focus on the present. Do not let the past or future control your thoughts. You cannot afford to waste your attention on past events such as a bad set or wasted time. Likewise, focusing on the future is fruitless. Because you have little control over the future, you will only miss out on the present training moment if you spend your time thinking about it.

Controlling your thoughts is not easy; it will take practice. You may find it helpful to use a focus word to get yourself back on track. For example, if you find that your thoughts are drifting away, you could use a word such as *concentrate* or *power* to return your attention to the present. Focusing on the present gives you the best opportunity to maintain intensity and develop your body. The faster you can return to a present focus, the better able you will be to concentrate for longer periods of time.

Self-Talk for Mood Adjustment

Bodybuilders need to train in a state of optimal arousal. That is, they should not be overaroused or underaroused. Self-talk can help you get into the optimal state of arousal during training and competition. For example, if you are angry or anxious, you must tell yourself to calm down and relax by using cue words that refocus your energy. Redirecting your energy will help keep you from wasting your energy on unproductive moods. If you are bored or fatigued, self-talk statements such as "I must renew my passion to get through this workout," or "I have what it takes and will give what it takes to build my body today" will restore the energy you need for intense training and competition.

Self-Talk for Muscle Confusion

In most sports, athletes rely on consistent practice to develop effective, habitual skill execution. The adage "practice makes perfect" has become the philosophy of coaches and athletes around the world. Consistent repetition of skills teaches the muscles and nervous system to execute physical movements as dependably and accurately as possible. This is a good thing, because it leads to automatic execution. Any good coach will tell you that performance suffers when an athlete has to think too much. Athletes who reach the highest levels of sport do so because they are able to execute skills flawlessly without thinking about it.

This flawless skill execution may be important to bodybuilders who perform choreographed routines in competition, but it has no place in the gym. It is critical that you be fully aware of what your muscles are doing during every set. Your movements cannot become so habitual that stagnancy results. Your muscles need to be in a constant state of confusion if you are going to see growth. If you simply go through the motions while you are working out, you might as well pack up your bags and go home. Your mind must continually challenge your body by remaining intensely focused on your task and thinking of ways to confuse your muscles into growth. Do not "zone out" during your workout, but rather use self-talk to help you "tune in" to what you are doing.

Self-Talk for Intensity Control

A typical workout lasts anywhere from 30 to 120 minutes, depending on your goals, the exercises involved, whether aerobic exercise is involved, and the availability of equipment. During a workout, you will have intense physical effort (reps and sets) followed by periods of recovery. As a bodybuilder, you must be able to control the amount of intensity, especially during sets. If your training sessions become boring or you become physically drained, you may question your reasons for bodybuilding. Self-coaching with focus words and positive statements can help you direct your effort levels and maintain intensity.

Muscular tone and growth come from discipline and the maintenance of intensity during workouts. If you are not experiencing success, it is likely

Mental Strength in the Face of Adversity: Victor Konovalov

Victor Konovalov is a three-time National Physique Committee (NPC) wheelchair overall champion (1996-1998) and was the first IFBB professional wheelchair bodybuilder. As a professional bodybuilder, Victor spends some of his time as a motivational speaker and has been a guest poser at the Mr. Olympia (1999-2000) and the NPC wheelchair nationals (1999). Strength training has helped him to overcome the emotional effects of his paralysis and has provided him with a unique perspective on the potential of the human body. Here are his thoughts on mental strength:

As a young soccer player, I established some good ground rules that have been a part of my life ever since. The first was commitment. I had to become responsible to myself and to other members of the team. The second rule was discipline. To become proficient and fully realize my potential, I had to practice a little more, try a bit harder, and be willing to take risks. In training, I have found that I have to constantly push myself through my thresholds and endure the pain. The third rule was sacrifice. I had to learn to establish priorities in my life and accept that some things would just have to come later.

Years later, when I broke my back and got into weight training to improve my health, I found that these traits were still with me. Almost instinctively, I pushed myself harder and harder. I wasn't content with merely working out. To this day, in my bodybuilding lifestyle, I continually compete against my own ability, testing it again and again so that I can be satisfied with the physical effort I have given in training.

I like to use imagery by envisioning my entire workout routine before I arrive at the gym. I see myself doing each exercise movement, and even challenge myself by mentally working through any sticking points. If a particular workout is going to require an intense focus, I usually begin thinking about it the day before. That way, when I enter the gym the next day, my focus and attention are immediately on my goal for that session. When I first arrive, I sometimes have to limit my social talking so that I can get right into my workout. I use that physical and mental energy for muscle-producing benefits instead. Finally, I find that if I think about the benefits I will derive from an intense workout, my attempts at reaching my goals become that much more effective.

that either your workouts lack intensity or your nutritional regimen is ineffective. In fact, the single factor that determines success in bodybuilding is a consistent pattern of high-intensity workouts. It is much better to have three to four high-intensity workouts of 30 to 40 minutes each than it is to have six moderate workouts of two hours each. It is extremely difficult to maintain high levels of intensity beyond 45 minutes in the gym. The good news is, less time can produce better results.

Eliminating Negative Self-Talk

There are two types of self-talk: negative and positive. While negative self-talk is common—"I'm such a loser," or "I wish I weren't such a weakling"—it can be particularly destructive for a bodybuilder.

But is negative self-talk any different from honestly rating your bodybuilding strengths and weaknesses? Certainly it is normal to evaluate yourself, identifying positive attributes as well as areas in need of improvement. In fact, it is absolutely necessary for optimal improvement. This becomes destructive when those target areas invade self-image, such as when you use your lack of strength or asymmetrical body as evidence that you are a "loser." When you have a negative self-image it is more likely that you will behave in ways that confirm those perceptions, thus proving to yourself and the rest of the world that you are indeed a loser.

Negative self-talk affects not only performance and self-image but also self-esteem. Remember, *self-image* is a term that describes the way you believe you look and present yourself to others. Self-esteem is an evaluative term that describes how you accept your self-image—positively or negatively. Bodybuilders who are excessively negative about themselves tend to

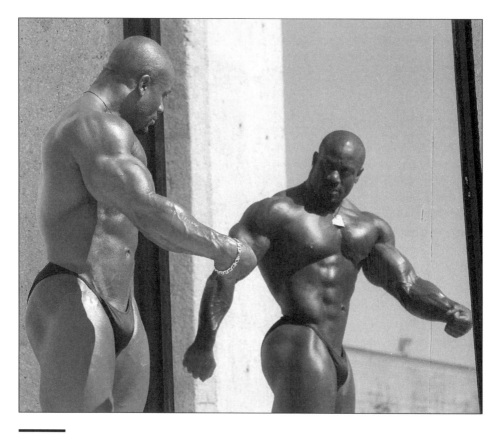

The way in which you talk to yourself plays an important role in determining your success.

drive themselves to depression. Unless chemically or hormonally induced, the fastest way out of a depressed state is consistent, continual, positive self-talk. For example, you should continuously remind yourself of your toned, muscular body; the improvements you have made since starting your bodybuilding program; and the bright future ahead.

The first step in eliminating negative self-talk is becoming aware of negative thoughts. Set out to change these self-esteem destroyers that live within you. Try putting a handful of toothpicks in your right pocket when you start your day. Each time you say something negative about yourself, move a toothpick from your right pocket to your left pocket. This way, you can see how many times a day you knock your self-esteem.

After the first day of toothpick transfer, sit down for 10 minutes and figure out what kinds of situations made you put yourself down. Was it the stress of work or school? Are you feeling a lot of pressure from your training partner, spouse, or friends about bodybuilding? Are you unhappy with your muscular size, definition, symmetry, or fitness level? Record your thoughts about the day into a log or journal. Writing them down will make them easier to change. As you look over your list, think about this: The problems you have with bodybuilding, work, school, or significant people in your life are not going to change by degrading yourself. Negative self-talk is only going to make the problems worse by lowering your self-esteem.

Now it is time to change that negative self-talk. The best technique for doing this is called "thought stopping." A process of replacing negative self-talk statements with positive self-talk statements, thought stopping includes three steps.

1. Identify the negative thought (this can include a mistake you made and now feel embarrassed about) or attitude.
2. Use a cue word (*wait* or *stop*) to stop the negative thought and clear your mind.
3. Replace the negative thought or attitude with a positive thought. For example, you might say "I'm never going to get as muscular as I want to be." "Stop." "I have already made a dramatic improvement in my body; with further practice, I will become more muscular and achieve the best body I can." Affirming statements about your body and about your life will not only enhance your self-esteem, but it also will allow you to train more effectively and enjoy the fruits of your hard work. Thought stopping can be extremely helpful in making this adjustment.

A Self-Coaching Plan

As you gain experience and your body becomes more developed, you will begin to take more responsibility for your own training and competitive attitude. You will begin to make decisions about bodybuilding that were once reserved for your training partner and personal trainer. You will decide whether you will work out, what your training program will consist of, what foods you will eat, whether you will take nutritional supplements, how much rest you need, and what your mental attitude will be during all facets of your training. Even if you have a personal trainer and/or training partner, you will have to coach yourself if you want to reach peak development. Bodybuilders unable to coach themselves become like robots, waiting for commands before they act.

Important Stages of a Workout

Every workout can be broken into four stages: workout preparation, during the workout, critical moments during the workout, and post-workout reflection. The self-coaching plan (exercise 6.1) that follows is based on these stages. Remember, use positive self-talk during each stage to ensure a successful workout. The following pages will guide you step-by-step through the stages of a workout and provide the opportunity to develop your own positive self-talk. Go through each stage carefully as you think about and prepare your self-coaching statements.

Self-Coaching Guidelines for Bodybuilders

Read through the following self-coaching guidelines, adapted from *Mental Skills for Swim Coaches*, and begin the process of becoming your own coach.[1]

- Turn negative thinking into positive thinking. Negative thinking is dysfunctional and ultimately leads to excessive states of worry. Bodybuilders who constantly worry about their performance will never be able to perform to their potential.
- Identify your self-talk patterns. To take control of, and possibly reverse, the way you talk to yourself, you must identify the strengths and weaknesses, the advantages and disadvantages, of your current self-talk.
- If you identify negative self-talk, be sure that you are willing to make necessary modifications.
- Positive self-talk is most effective when it is spontaneous and part of your everyday language. Work positive affirmations into your self-talk first, then add specifics to give it truer meaning.
- Think, rethink, read, and reread your positive self-coaching statements until they become part of you. Once they become ingrained, you will find that your old way of thinking will be less and less evident in your life.
- Remember that you will make mistakes. No one is perfect. Focus your attention on giving 100 percent effort every time you perform, and know that your hard work and skills will come through more often than not.

Exercise 6.1 | Self-Coaching Plan

STAGE 1: WORKOUT PREPARATION

1. Do not think that you are helpless or weak. Develop self-coaching statements that will help you change this thinking before the workout begins. Use these statements to get started on making your own.
   - "I can do this workout. Let me actively prepare."
   - "I must think about what I can do to deal with this. I will think about a plan for this workout."
   - "This is my favorite part of the day. What new way can I challenge my quads during my workout?"

Add other statements that will reverse a helpless or weak attitude.

_____

_____

_____

2. Keep a positive attitude. Practice thought stopping to transform negative attitudes into positive ones. Here are some self-talk statements you could use:
   - "I will remain positive during this workout. My feelings of fear are my body's way of getting ready for a big lift."
   - "What mental strategies can I use to help me get over my concerns or fears?"
   - "Being tired is no reason to have a bad workout. I am a bodybuilder and I need to train. I can feel the energy moving through my muscles when I breathe deeply and relax."

Add other statements that will help you stay positive.

_____

_____

_____

STAGE 2: DURING THE WORKOUT

3. During the workout, you will need to be mentally focused on tasks, in an optimal state of arousal, and in a positive frame of mind. Use the mental strategies presented throughout this book, switching strategies as

(continued)

129

necessary and using self-coaching statements to direct your focus. Remember, you are your own coach now.

Here are examples of self-coaching statements.

- "Okay, I'm being distracted by other people in the gym. That means I should take some slow, deep breaths and focus on what is important."

- "I must stop these negative thoughts and replace them with positive ones. I do belong here, and when I train with intensity, I am able to get awesome results."

- "I am becoming fatigued as the workout wears on. Wait! I'll repeat the word *power* to energize me and help me to complete this workout with enthusiasm and energy."

- "Relax. Just breathe deeply and relax. I am more than capable of pushing myself through this workout with passion and intensity."

- "Concentrate. I will say *force* while I continue to breathe in a controlled manner during relaxation. This will keep me in an optimal state of arousal and performance."

- "I won't think about my physical exhaustion. I will focus my attention on how strong I am and how I am going to use my powerful muscles and breathing to complete these sets."

Add other statements that you can say to yourself to stay focused.

_____

_____

_____

4. In chapter 10, you will learn more mental strategies to make your workouts more effective, such as specific breathing techniques (ratio or complete breathing) and developing body awareness. Once you have read chapter 10, complete your list of self-coaching statements in the space provided. Also use the imagery, relaxation, and mental skills techniques discussed earlier in this book.

_____

_____

_____

_____

_____

STAGE 3: CRITICAL MOMENTS IN THE WORKOUT

5. Almost always, you will have critical moments during a workout, those times when you must consciously decide whether to persevere or quit. For example, your partner may want to stop training or may be making it difficult for you to focus. Critical moments also happen on the individual level, such as when you have made a mistake in a set or sheer exhaustion renders you unable to complete the set. You may start to feel weak or be excessively hard on yourself for letting your partner, and yourself, down. It is during these times that positive self-coaching statements become invaluable.

Some examples of positive self-coaching statements:

- "Come on! This is my last set. I am going to forget that last set and focus on the next one. I am going to use all my strength and will to finish strong."
- "If I lose my focus, I will not let it get me down. I will think positively for the rest of the workout. I will be intense for the remaining sets."
- "I have trained hard all year and I know that I can do this. I just need to dig a little deeper and have a better attitude. I will not give up on myself or my training partner. I will strive to be the best bodybuilder I can be."

Add some other positive self-coaching statements.

_____

_____

_____

6. When you find yourself succumbing to negative thoughts or feelings, make an effort to stop them. Substitute positive self-coaching to get you back on the right track. The following self-coaching statements will get you started.

- "This workout is not going like I had planned. I can't take anymore—No, wait a minute. I will not make things worse than they really are. I'll concentrate on my breathing and center my thoughts on what I have control over."
- "I am lifting terribly. Things are falling apart!—Stop. Stop thinking that. Relax. It is better to focus my attention on something else. Take a few deep breaths and regain control. . . . Good."
- "There's no use. I should just quit bodybuilding—Hold on! Thinking like that is crazy. Anyone can have a bad workout. That is no reason to quit. I can do this. I am capable. OK, take a deep breath and get your thoughts back on track."

(continued)

Add more self-coaching statements that will help you stay positive during critical moments in the workout.

_____

_____

_____

_____

_____

STAGE 4: POST-WORKOUT REFLECTION

7. At first, you may have difficulty speaking to yourself positively. Do not lose heart if you have a long history of negative thoughts and self-talk. Positive self-coaching will take practice, especially in difficult and stressful situations. You deserve a pat on the back for having tried. If you have been able to be even a little more positive, you should feel proud. Take this opportunity to practice positive self-coaching by complimenting yourself on your effort, if not your progress. The following are some examples:

   • "I knew hard work could carry me through the workout. Sure, I gave up on some sets, but overall I lifted very well. I am getting better all the time. I am proud of myself."

   • "I did it! I was able to stay positive during my workout and I lifted well. It is reassuring to know that I can coach myself through the program I have worked hard all year to develop. I know that I can coach myself through future workouts."

   • "I thought my training partner was going to quit, but I am happy with the effort he put in."

Add your own positive reflection statements here.

_____

_____

_____

_____

_____

- Plan to spend time each day coaching yourself through your training program, nutritional regimen, and lifestyle patterns. Then spend some time every night reviewing how you did that day and rehearsing your positive self-coaching statements for the next day.

Attributional Style

At every level of competitive sport, there are athletes who win and there are athletes who lose. Invariably, there are many more losers than winners. Each year, only one team wins the Super Bowl, and only one tennis player wins the U.S. Open (in each category). In the Boston Marathon, out of the thousands who participate, only one male and one female are crowned the champions. The same is true in amateur bodybuilding. Only one person is declared the winner in each weight division and only one overall champion is declared among division winners. Both winning and losing are part of the sport experience, and unfortunately, losing is the more common of the two.

In your bodybuilding program over the years, you will have successes (such as increasing the strength of deltoids) and you will have failures (such as gaining 10 pounds of body fat). For each of your failures and successes, you will undoubtedly have at least one explanation. And if you are like most people, you will attempt to accept your successes and excuse your failures.

Athletes and coaches attribute losing to many reasons, ranging from bad weather or officiating to a lack of ability or effort. Reasons for winning vary to the same degree as those for losing. Because there are so many losers and so few winners in sport, it is important that athletes redefine their notions of success and failure. There must be more to success in bodybuilding than winning a competition or looking like the bodybuilders in muscle magazines. Success can also include placing higher in a competition, bench pressing 200 pounds for the first time, and being able to see results after sticking with your nutritional program. *Success* and *failure* will mean different things for different people, so you must come up with your own measure.

Whatever people attribute their success or failure to, it is an important psychological consideration, called "attributional style." Your attributional style is important to your future success as a bodybuilder. Indeed, it dictates how you approach training and determines the strength of your commitment to the bodybuilding lifestyle. For example, by attributing a competition win to biased judges, you are indicating that you believe yourself incapable of winning without them. This view is a defeatist approach to bodybuilding and will have a detrimental effect on your level of motivation for future training and competition. By attributing that win to hard work and personal effort, on the other hand, you are indicating that you believe yourself capable of success and improvement.

People attribute success and failure according to their own biases. The three major biases that affect attributional style are informational, perceptual, and motivational.

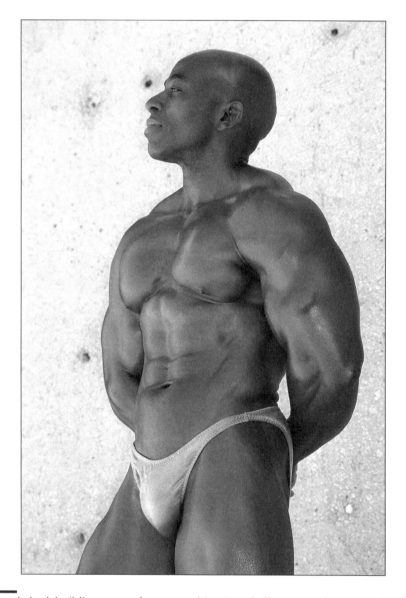

Success in bodybuilding comes from a combination of effort, commitment, and genetics.

Informational Biases

As their label suggests, informational biases stem from information, including information you know about yourself or others as well as information others know about you. For example, you may enter a competition in which you know little about the opposition and the opposition knows little about you. You may attribute a competitor's excellent physique to genetics, when the truth is that he or she excelled through hard work and proper nutrition. Misunderstandings of motives and behaviors are commonplace in situations where a lack of information leads to an incomplete assessment.

Perceptual Biases

Perceptual biases result because it is difficult to observe yourself. The inability to observe yourself, makes it difficult to know yourself objectively. For example, your perception of how you look will likely differ from how others see you, because you cannot see your every move in the gym or on stage. Onlookers, however, can see exactly how you behave.

   If you have ever recorded your voice on a cassette recorder and been surprised at the sound of your voice when you played back the cassette, you understand the concept of perceptual bias. Your perception of how you sound is inaccurate, because you are hearing yourself through your own ears and not through the ears of those around you. In the same way, bodybuilders are perceptually biased about their own body strengths and weaknesses. Bodybuilders sometimes see the cause of failure as being out of their control—they got stuck with faulty genes, bad luck, poor advice, or bad judging—but more often than not, this is simply a perceptual bias at work.

Motivational Biases

Motivational biases can affect the way bodybuilders view the road to success. Many see success as the result of personal ability and effort, and see failure as the result of factors beyond their control. Being aware of what motivates you to train and compete as a bodybuilder is essential if you want to maximize your potential.

   Exercise 6.2 will help you become aware of your personal biases and how they affect your definitions of *success* and *failure*. After you answer the questions, take a few moments to reflect on your explanations about bodybuilding successes and failures. Understanding your attributional biases and the way you arrive at them is essential if you want to adjust them later on.

Explanatory Style

In his book *Learned Optimism,* Martin Seligman maintains that different people have different ways of explaining setbacks in their lives. Some people automatically attribute failure to themselves, while others see failure as a temporary setback and not really due to anything within themselves. Seligman calls explaining events in this way "explanatory style." [2]

   Explanatory style, illustrated in figure 6.1, is either optimistic or pessimistic. Like the maxim "you attract more bees with honey than with vinegar," success is more likely to follow optimism than pessimism.

Permanent Versus Temporary

Permanence is one of the ways people view success and failure, specifically, whether they view that failure or success as enduring or short lived. People

Exercise 6.2   Attribution Questions

- Do you have all the necessary information to make an accurate judgment about other bodybuilders?

- Have you asked at least three informed people for their opinion of your body?

- Do you view success in bodybuilding as a result of your genetics, intensity of training, or commitment to the bodybuilding lifestyle?

- Do you view failure in bodybuilding as a result of things out of your control, such as genetics, bad officiating, or an unsuitable place to train?

- Do you simply need to increase your training effort to improve your body, or are you already reaching your genetic potential?

who view life pessimistically do not typically persist after a disappointing performance, believing that the cause of the poor performance is permanent. Pessimists rarely stick with a challenging task, adopting a defeatist attitude that leaves them discouraged about their chance for future success. Even with a good performance, pessimists still believe their good fortune is temporary and will not last for any significant period of time.

Optimists view life from a different perspective. They bounce back from poor performances, called *reboundability,* and persist in the face of adversity, believing the cause to be temporary. To the optimistic person, good performances are permanent and will last for a long time. An optimistic bodybuilder is able to rebound quickly from bad workouts or minor injuries that take them away from the gym.

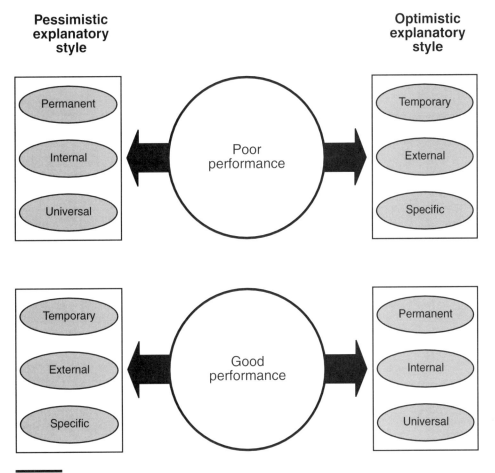

Figure 6.1 Explanatory style.

Adapted from Seligman 1990.

Specific Versus Universal

Individuals respond differently to positive and negative occurrences and the way in which they allow those occurrences to infiltrate other areas of their lives. Pessimists give up when they are disappointed and use universal explanations to explain poor performance. A universal explanation extends beyond the sport setting into other areas of life. For example, if dissatisfied with their training performance, pessimistic bodybuilders may not only view their training as a failure but perceive they are also failures in other areas of their lives. Pessimistic bodybuilders typically view good perfor-

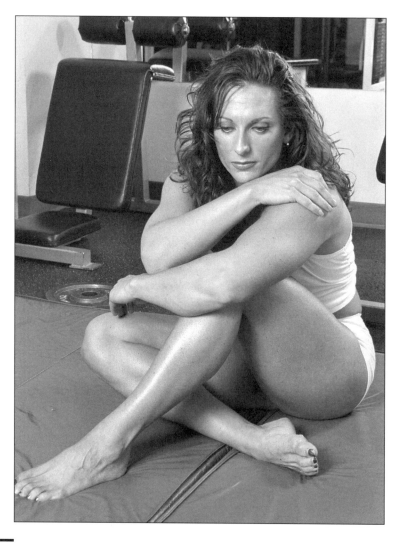

Believing in yourself and having an optimistic outlook will enhance your bodybuilding experience.

mance as specific to the sport of bodybuilding. Thus, success in bodybuilding has little carryover into other areas.

Optimists, on the other hand, explain failure specifically and save the universal explanation for success. For optimistic bodybuilders, positive experiences in the gym or during competition are extended. Success in bodybuilding leads them to believe that they can be successful in other areas of life.

Internal Versus External

The final characteristic of explanatory style refers to whether a person internalizes failure or success, that is, whether a person attributes success or failure in bodybuilding to personal causes. Pessimists consistently blame themselves for bad things they have little or no control over, such as faulty gym equipment. Bodybuilders who continually accept blame for a poor performance, even if they had no control over the situation, will ultimately believe that they are failures. Good performances, on the other hand, are externalized by pessimists to the point that they do not take any credit for success.

Conversely, optimistic bodybuilders are able to assess a situation, identifying those things they had control over and those things they did not. Good performances are internalized by optimists, who are all too happy to take credit for their success and trust that they will be able to perform well again in the future.

The ABCs of Developing an Optimistic Explanatory Style

It is extremely important that bodybuilders have an optimistic outlook, both in their sport and on life in general. Exercise 6.3 will assist you in developing an optimistic explanatory style. Make sure that you go through each of the steps in the order they are shown.

"Know thyself and coach thyself." It is a great motto for every bodybuilder. In the sport of bodybuilding, you will rely on the abilities and knowledge of others to develop your body, but when it comes down to the crunch, you will have to rely on yourself: your internal and external strengths and skills. Although the emphasis in bodybuilding is often on working out, working within is just as—if not more—important. Indeed, the greater the power of your mental skills, the easier it will be for you to train with a level of intensity that promotes muscle growth and strength.

Exercise 6.3 | Developing an Optimistic Explanatory Style

Every athlete has a characteristic pattern of explaining failure and success in sport. This exercise is intended to help you determine your current explanatory style for events of adversity. Once you know your current explanatory style you will be able to make any necessary adjustments.

Adversity

While undesirable, certainly, poor performance is the perfect opportunity for you to develop as a bodybuilder. The presence of adversity provides an excellent training ground for the development of an optimistic explanatory style. In the space provided, record adverse events as they occur or reflect back on some adverse circumstances you have encountered within your season or career.

Adverse event #1 _____

Adverse event #2 _____

Adverse event #3 _____

Adverse event #4 _____

Belief

For each adversity, record your beliefs about that specific event. Try to distinguish between your thoughts and feelings. Thoughts are your beliefs about the event. Feelings are your reactions to those beliefs or to the event itself. For example, you might *believe* you lost a competition because your abdominal section is weak, but your *feelings* would be frustration or anger. Record your beliefs in this section and record your feelings in the next section, Consequences.

Adverse event #1

Beliefs: _____

Adverse event #2

Beliefs: _____

Adverse event #3

Beliefs: _____

Adverse event #4

Beliefs: _____

Analyze your beliefs. Are they permanent? How pervasive are they? Have you personalized them?

Consequences

For each belief, note your specific feelings and actions, if any. Did you feel sad? Happy? Anxious? Remember that feelings are your reactions to your beliefs or to the event itself. Look for links between your beliefs and their consequences.

Adverse event #1

*Beliefs:*_____

*Feelings:*_____

Adverse event #2

*Beliefs:*_____

*Feelings:*_____

Adverse event #3

*Beliefs:*_____

*Feelings:*_____

Adverse event #4

*Beliefs:*_____

*Feelings:*_____

Disputation

Now that you have completed the Beliefs and Consequences section, you may have found that you have a pessimistic explanatory style, which leads to negative consequences. If so, it is time to learn to dispute those negative, pessimistic beliefs.

Learn to argue with yourself when your explanatory style is self-destructive. In other words, convince yourself that your pessimism is going to hurt your body development, and make a change as soon as possible. This is a good time to use thought stopping to change your current thinking into something more positive. The more you change your negative outlook, the more positive it will become in the future. In the future, minor negatives are going to be that much easier to change when a positive explanatory style is the norm.

Energization

In addition to a more positive outlook, the result of continual disputation of a negative or pessimistic explanatory style is increased energy and motivation. In other words, you will spend more of your mental energy focused on improving your body rather than speaking negatively to yourself and others. When you take on a more positive approach to your training, nutritional habits, and lifestyle, you will become an energized bodybuilder who is able to avoid debilitating anxiety.

CHAPTER 7

Pushing the Intensity Barrier

"Come on, make it hurt." "No pain, no gain." "Push through the pain." These and similar statements are heard in bodybuilding gyms across the world. Is there any truth to them? Is pain essential for a good workout? The secret to success in bodybuilding is performing lifts with enough intensity to increase strength and muscular size. So, to answer the question, it is essential that most of your workouts are performed with great intensity. There are times when the intensity level will be so high that you will likely experience some pain.

What Is Intensity?

Intensity can be thought of as the application of maximum physical effort to a motor skill. This includes the effort that is required for a successful bodybuilding program. However, you must first understand and be able to execute proper lifting techniques before you start concentrating on effort. Focusing on technique prevents both injury and subsequent disappointment. Once you have developed proper lifting techniques, preferably to an intermediate level, then you are ready to start increasing your effort.

High-intensity training is going all out, no less than all out. It is about taking each set to the absolute limit and making a commitment to correct bad habits such as resting excessively between sets, spending an inordinate amount of time posing in the mirror or socializing, and simply going through the motions. High-intensity training is not easy. It involves serious muscular effort to pull or push as hard as you possibly can, especially during the final reps of a set. Bodybuilders in high-intensity training often reach physical exhaustion. That is, they get to the point where their muscles will work no more. This momentary muscular failure in the final reps of a set should be a goal for every high-intensity workout.

Performing an exercise to the point of physical failure is difficult, both from a physiological and a psychological perspective. The muscles are exhausted and being filled with lactic acid, which causes the burning sensation, and the mind would rather give up than push ahead. Pushing through is not easy, but it is necessary for maximum growth. When you exert maximum effort, your body sends a signal to your muscles to grow stronger and larger to ensure that similar stress will be tolerable in the future. Of course, you trick your muscles by increasing the load the next time you work out. High-intensity training becomes a game of breakdown and buildup.

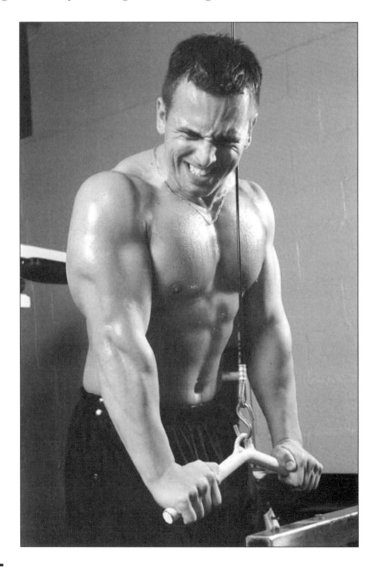

Intensity leads to momentary muscular failure and results in maximum growth.

You break down the muscle, let it build back up during rest, and then break it down again, going on and on until you reach your bodybuilding potential.

Of course, you will also need to integrate some easy weeks and workouts in your program to achieve optimum muscular growth. Nevertheless, the basic rule in bodybuilding is to look for ways to increase the intensity of your exercise, not make it easier. This is achieved by increasing reps or sets, decreasing rest periods, using supersets or tri-sets, or coming up with creative ways to isolate a muscle group. High-intensity exercise may not be as enjoyable as easy exercise, but the rewards are significantly more enjoyable.

Here is a word of caution: do not make the mistake of confusing "high intensity" with length of time or number of sets. A novice bodybuilder who was excited about getting big once told me that he intended to train six days a week for two hours each day, or 12 hours per week. He wanted to impress me with that information, but I was not impressed. I knew that most of his time would be wasted, because it would be impossible for him to maintain high intensity for that length of time. High-intensity exercise must be brief. Workouts do not need to be any longer than 45 minutes after warm-up. Any longer than that simply means that the intensity level is not high enough during sets or that rest periods are too long.

Pain and Intensity

Pain is natural in every athletic experience, whether track and field, swimming, football, volleyball, or boxing. Bill Koch, a silver medalist in the 30K cross-country ski event at the 1976 Olympics, said that 90 percent of his success had to do with his ability to tolerate pain.[1] Greg LeMond, three-time winner of the Tour de France, the most grueling race in sport history, said this about cycling: "... the best climbers are those ... who can stand the most pain. ... in pro cycling everything hurts, but you just ride through it."[2] While the sports of bodybuilding and cycling differ dramatically, the necessity of pain tolerance is the same in both. Every bodybuilder, from the beginner to the most successful competitor, can benefit from understanding how pain affects the workout session and how to overcome its debilitating effects.

The capacity to tolerate pain is among the most important features of bodybuilding success. Not all bodybuilders experience pain in the same way, however. The perception of pain is dependent on physiological, psychological, environmental, and situational factors. It is therefore important that you have a good understanding of your pain-management skills if you are to improve your ability to tolerate pain. The role that mental skills play in the perception and tolerance of pain is explained in figure 7.1.

Pain Mechanisms

The gate-control theory of pain, updated by Melzack and Wall in 1988, proposes that a neural mechanism in the spinal cord acts like a gate,

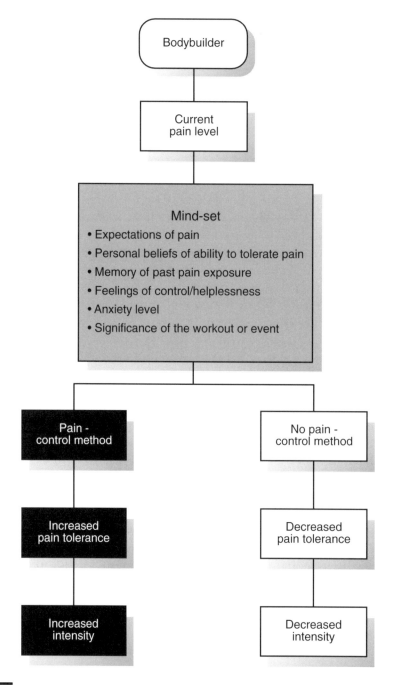

Figure 7.1 Mind-set and the debilitating effects of training pain.

controlling the flow of nerve impulses from peripheral fibers to the central nervous system. The degree to which the flow of nerve impulses increases or decreases is regulated by the afferent nerve fibers and by influences from the higher brain centers. When the amount of information passing through the gates exceeds a critical level, it activates three different neural areas. Each neural area is responsible for a distinct aspect of the pain experience.[3]

These three neural areas, or systems—the sensory-discriminative system, the motivational-affective system, and the cognitive-evaluative system—carry information to the brain. The sensory-discriminative system carries information about the location and intensity of the stimulation. The motivational-affective system carries information about the aversive qualities of the pain and stimulates the "fight or flight" response. The cognitive-evaluative system interprets the pain experience. These three systems work together with the central control process and the brain to determine the appropriate psychological response to a painful stimulus

So what does all of this have to do with bodybuilding? Prior to the development of the gate-control theory, scientists believed that people were either born with pain tolerance or were not, and that no one could improve that predetermined pain tolerance. Current research shows that the way people think about pain and the way they choose to deal with that pain can have a tremendous impact on whether they can tolerate it. Indeed, it has been shown that bodybuilders who use pain-control methods, such as relaxation, imagery, self-coaching, and so on, are able to tolerate higher levels of pain during a workout and thus develop more muscle.

According to the gate-control theory, modification of such cognitive processes as positive thinking and directed focus can reduce perceived pain. In other words, anxiety, attention, and past experience can affect the sensation of pain. Maladaptive activities, including arousal and anxiety, must be identified and changed before the physiology responsible for pain perception is activated. The short of it is, your mind plays a crucial role in reducing and increasing the experience of pain.

Pain has a distinctly unpleasant quality. It can be overwhelming, demand immediate attention, disrupt ongoing behavior and thought, and motivate you to stop whatever you are doing as quickly as possible. This is why some bodybuilders seem to have higher or lower levels of pain tolerance than others. This is why some bodybuilders can train with greater intensity than others. The ability to tolerate pain is largely dependent on how you perceive the pain experience.

In every moment of training, your brain is aware of both your body and the surrounding environment. As it receives each new stimulus, the brain identifies, organizes, and evaluates it. In the case of physical discomfort, this process is called "pain perception." Your reaction to pain can be explained largely by your level of anxiety, previous experience with intense training, attitude, and the coping skills you have available to you.

Research shows that bodybuilders form a pattern of response to the pain or burn that comes with difficult training sets. That response pattern then determines their attitude and response to future sets and workouts. Since pain is most often associated with distress, it is likely that most people react to pain with a distress pattern. In the case of bodybuilding, if you experience

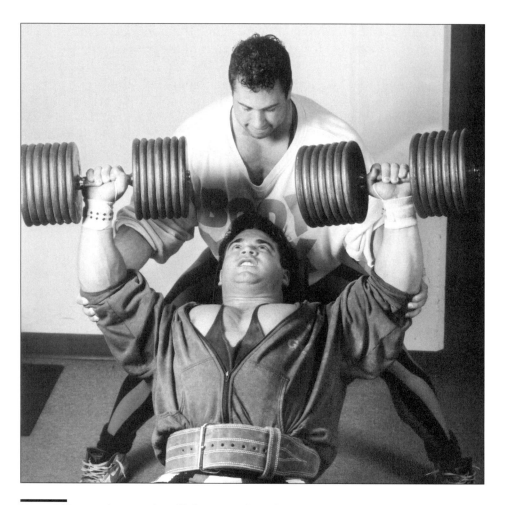

Your ability to tolerate pain will determine how far you can push your body.

pain during a workout, you will likely see it as distressful and choose to quit the exercise. The key, then, is to focus not on the emotional and distressing aspects but rather on the sensory qualities of pain. This will make it easier to see the contribution that pain makes to overall muscle growth.

You see, pain tolerance goes far beyond your muscular size, strength, or physiological condition. Frankly, your ability to tolerate pain has very little to do with your body. The ability to tolerate pain while training has more to do with your mind. Surely you have had workouts when you could not seem to break through the intensity barrier, no matter how hard you tried, and other workouts when you were Captain Pain Tolerance. You did not lose strength overnight, nor did you lose muscular size. No, you just responded to the set differently than you did the time before.

Bodybuilding and Pain

For your workouts to be most productive, you must maintain a high level of intensity throughout, increasing the amount of blood flow to each working muscle. This is the "pump" that many bodybuilders experience after each workout. To experience this "pump," you will no doubt encounter a corresponding level of physical pain. In fact, the more pain you experience while working the muscle, the greater the "pump."

Every experienced bodybuilder recognizes that pain is a necessary part of a successful workout, but can too much pain be damaging or cause injury? Most sport coaches and weightlifting instructors agree that it is not really a question of how much pain, but rather the type and location of the pain. If you feel a dull, burning pain in the "belly" of the working muscle, you can assume that the exercise is safe and will not cause injury. This type of pain is fatigue related, an uncomfortable but natural part of the weightlifting experience. On the other hand, if you feel a sharp, shooting pain in the joint (such as in the elbows, knees, shoulders), you should stop immediately. This type of pain is injury related and may cause damage to the connective tissues, such as ligaments or tendons.

While achieving optimal results means pushing through fatigue-related pain during a workout, it is foolish to push through injury-related pain. Bodybuilding injuries require long periods of recovery and time away from training, which will be detrimental to muscular strength and size in the long run.

Bodybuilders use different techniques to increase the intensity and further fatigue the muscles, including supersets, tri-sets, giant sets, forced reps, pre-exhaustion, "cheating," and training to failure, among others. While all of these techniques are effective in maintaining intensity, they are also highly painful. It is virtually impossible to have high-intensity, muscle-building workouts without high levels of physical discomfort. It would be like trying to play baseball without a bat, or tennis without a racket. To overcome the pain associated with high-intensity workouts, effective bodybuilders use their mental skills to push through difficult workouts to achieve their bodybuilding goals.

Pain Tolerance

Unique to every bodybuilder, pain perception can affect the intensity level of your workout. Take the case of one bodybuilder: "I get physically tired and my muscles get sore," he says. "I try to get myself psyched up for the workout, but when my muscles hurt, I'll take it easy until the physical pain is gone before I'll push myself hard in weight training again." This athlete has allowed his pain to dictate his intensity level. When the pain becomes too much to handle, he decreases the intensity of his workouts, which will only result in less than optimal results. Another bodybuilder says, "Physically,

Intensity Revisited: Dan Wagman

Dan Wagman, PhD, CSCS, has won an International Powerlifting Federation (IPF) and American Powerlifting Federation world title, an IPF silver medal, two IPF bronze medals, and three U.S. Powerlifting Federation national championships. Dan has set national and world (IPF) records in the bench press and recorded the second-highest strict curl in the U.S. Strict Curl Association, where he is also recognized as a national champion. Drawing from his extensive experience as a strength athlete, Dan shares the following thoughts on training and intensity:

One of the most appealing aspects of strength sport is the high level of intensity packed into a few seconds of activity. Nothing feels better than setting up to lift a bar bent under a load never lifted before, feeling your body nearly buckle under the strain, then explosively and successfully lifting the weight through a complete range of motion. Like most athletes, I believe that hard work and persistence yield results. Training intensity should be held in the highest regard by strength athletes. While training intensity is the key to success, however, measured intensity will take you even farther. The bottom line: train too hard for too long, and you'll burn out.

In 1991, I experienced firsthand how intensity can be taken too far, manifesting itself physically and psychologically. I had forced myself to stick with my training weights in preparation for the world championships. I say "forced" because for some reason I didn't feel like training. I pushed myself hard and was able to make my training weights, but as training progressed, I experienced an ever-increasing level of self-doubt: Why were the weights so heavy? What the heck was I doing wrong? Was I really made for this?

When it came right down to it, I needed a 700-pound dead lift for the gold, a weight I lifted in training a week earlier. I gave it a monstrous effort, my muscles screaming under the load and my tendons quivering under the strain, yet I was unable to raise the bar beyond my knees. I ended up with a bronze medal, finding no satisfaction with that accomplishment. I had tried so hard. Why didn't my muscles follow my command? My level of self-doubt was at an all-time high. On the flight back to the States, I had time to reflect. I realized that my body was totally spent after competing in seven major competitions in two years. It was just too much. No wonder I disliked training and my lifts came so close to crushing me.

After delving deeply into training science, I realized that it is impossible to separate psychology from physiology. An elite strength athlete must learn to effectively address both the mind and body with a balanced and measured approach. You must train hard, but at the same time you must control your training intensity to match the level of your psyche.

every muscle feels sore and fatigued. They just hurt. When I really start to feel the pain in my muscles, I tell myself to keep going and force myself to push through hard on every rep and set." This bodybuilder also experiences high levels of pain during his workouts, but he is determined to maintain a high level of intensity, regardless of the pain.

Bodybuilders with lower levels of pain tolerance tend to train less often and for shorter periods of time than bodybuilders with higher levels of pain tolerance. Keeping in mind the importance of muscle recuperation, it is essential that you maintain consistency in both workout frequency and duration. Workouts of high physical intensity provide an easy excuse for missing the next workout or decreasing the amount of time spent in the gym. Statements like "My last workout was hard, so today I will shorten the workout," or "I am only going to train two times per week because the workouts are physically draining," are common among bodybuilders who are unable to tolerate high levels of pain.

Once you begin to use pain as an excuse for limiting the frequency or duration of regular workout sessions, you are a just a small step away from quitting your training program altogether. Your likelihood of maintaining an effective training program depends on two factors: your ability to handle the pain of high-intensity workouts and whether you see positive results from your workouts. Because bodybuilders with low pain tolerance typically opt for low-intensity workouts, not to mention fewer and shorter workouts, they tend to see fewer results, which leads to disappointment and eventually quitting their training altogether. The key to achieving positive results is to train with high intensity, to effectively manage the pain, and then to rest, allowing for full recovery between workouts.

Bodybuilders who use coping skills to manage their pain improve their performance dramatically. This has been shown over and over in various studies on pain tolerance and sport. Of course, the first step in pain management is identifying your level of pain tolerance and how it affects your workouts. Exercise 7.1 will help you do just that.

Now that you have a better idea of the way you experience and manage pain, it is time to change your perception of pain. A positive mind-set is an essential, integral part of effective bodybuilding. With the right mental skills, you can control your pain and lessen its effects. As discussed earlier in this book, athletes who demonstrate a higher level of pain tolerance in most situations achieve a higher level of performance than athletes with a lower level of pain tolerance. Moreover, athletes who push themselves to their cognitive limits actually perceive themselves as more satisfied with both the process and the result.

Pain Control

One of the most effective methods of pain control is avoiding unnecessary tension in the muscles during a workout, particularly tension in muscles that

Exercise 7.1 How Is Your Pain Tolerance?

1. Describe the pain you typically feel during a workout.

   _____

   _____

   _____

2. When does pain occur? Is it intermittent or continuous during training sessions?

   _____

   _____

   _____

3. What exercises are you unable to do because of physical discomfort?

   _____

   _____

   _____

4. What, if anything, do you do to relieve the pain? Do certain actions, thoughts, or feelings make the pain worse?

   _____

   _____

   _____

5. Does the pain interfere with your bodybuilding enjoyment? What emotions do you feel when you are experiencing pain in training?

   _____

   _____

   _____

6. Comment on your ability to tolerate physical discomfort in workouts. Are you confident in your level of pain tolerance?

   _____

   _____

   _____

are not working. Bodybuilders must learn how to relax the non working muscles so that they can differentiate between pain signals related to muscle strength and growth and pain signals that are not. Pain that occurs in the belly of the working muscle is likely related to muscle growth. Pain experienced in the joints or the connective tissues is unrelated to muscle growth and may be an indication of an ensuing injury.

Relaxation

While it may seem that relaxation and high intensity are incompatible, this is not the case. To effectively isolate signals from working muscles, the rest of the body must be relaxed. Relaxation also facilitates recovery between sets and workouts, promotes the onset of sleep, and may even relieve undesirable muscular tension such as headaches or lower back aches.

The advantages of relaxation training are (1) anyone can learn it, and (2) most people will see an improvement within two to three weeks of regular practice. Relaxation skills must be practiced on a regular basis, just like any other sport skill. During the learning process, it is best to practice relaxation away from the gym. Once you develop your relaxation skills, you can introduce them into your workouts.

The relaxation techniques that are most applicable to reducing pain in bodybuilding are the "mind-to-muscle" techniques. These rely on meditation and/or mental imagery. Mind-to-muscle relaxation first relaxes the mind, which results in physical relaxation. One of the most useful mind-to-muscle techniques for athletes is Benson's Relaxation Response (discussed in chapter 10). *Relaxation response* refers to the capacity of the body to enter a special relaxation state, characterized by lower heart and breathing rates, a decrease in blood pressure, slower brain waves, and an overall reduction in the speed of metabolism. The changes produced by the relaxation response can counteract the discomfort of physical exertion and pain. Benson's Relaxation Response can be done in bed, in the car, at school or work, and during a workout—in short, it can be done anywhere and at any time of day.

Imagery

Your thoughts, expectations, and ideas can dramatically affect the way you feel and behave. A faulty mind-set about pain during a workout can lead to feelings of nervousness, worry, increased pain, and ultimately failure. On the other hand, a positive mind-set can lead to relaxation, self-confidence, and decreased pain. This is where imagery comes in.

Imagery strategies such as dissociation and association can be used to enhance pain tolerance and strength in specific muscle groups. Dissociation is the process of focusing your attention away from the pain, using distractions that are either internal (mental arithmetic, counting, or singing a song) or external (listening to music or watching videos). Association involves

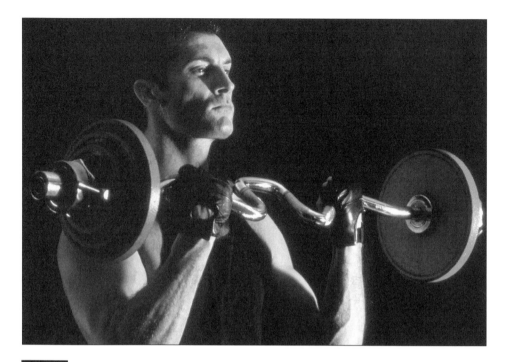

Controlling pain with a positive mind-set and the use of imagery are keys to success in bodybuilding.

focusing on bodily sensations, maintaining performance-related physical awareness, or changing the perception of the pain.

Since bodybuilders have a deep appreciation of the relationship between pain and strength training, it is likely that association techniques will be the most effective. Nevertheless, it is always a good idea to add a number of different imagery and mental skills to your repertoire. Following are six different techniques. Practice each one at home a few times, and then choose one or two of the best ones that you can use during workouts.

1. Imaginative inattention. This technique involves ignoring the pain by evoking images that are incompatible with the pain experience. For example, imagine yourself going to the beach or swimming in the crystal-blue waters of Hawaii. Thinking about a pleasurable experience takes your mind off the pain in your working muscles.

2. Imaginative transformation of pain. This technique involves acknowledging the pain but interpreting it as trivial or unreal. I once met a bodybuilder who told me that whenever he experienced pain in training, he would simply dismiss it as a small nuisance. For example, when you are in pain, try transforming it by saying, "This pain is nothing," or "I have experienced worse pain." Then push through your set as if it did not hurt too badly.

3. Imaginative transformation of context. Like you do with imaginative transformation of pain, you acknowledge the pain in imaginative transfor-

mation of context, but this time you transform the setting. For example, you may picture yourself as James Bond being shot in the leg while running away from terrorists, or you may imagine that the pain in your biceps is a knife wound you incurred while protecting your family from an attacker.

4. External attention diversion. This technique involves diverting your attention from the pain to some physical characteristic of the environment that has nothing to do with the actual exercise. For example, you may look at yourself in the mirror, focus on a particular piece of equipment in the gym, or look out the window. In fact, one of the reasons that gyms have a lot of mirrors and windows is to divert people's attention from the pain of workouts.

5. Internal attention diversion. As with external attention diversion, this technique involves diverting your attention from the pain, but with internal attention diversion, you focus on your thoughts, going "inside your head." For example, you may think of a favorite song, count backward from 1,000 by 7s, design a new room for your house, and so on. Any internal mental activity that distracts you from the pain will be effective.

6. Somatization. A common technique used by bodybuilders, somatization involves focusing on the part of the body receiving intense stimulation but in a detached manner. While doing a standing biceps curl, you would analyze the physical sensations you experience. Somatization involves thinking about the muscle, connective tissue, and bone activity that make the movement possible. This technique is excellent for muscle isolation.

With the exception of external attention diversion, every one of the above techniques relies on your ability to imagine and visualize. Use exercise 7.2 to practice your imagery skills and determine which imagery technique is most effective for managing your pain. Once you know which imagery technique(s) you prefer, you can begin to lessen the pain of high-intensity workouts.

Self-Coaching

If you are like most bodybuilders, you do not have a training coach. Most bodybuilders coach themselves. It is essential to coach yourself through difficult sets in the same way that a training coach would. Self-coaching involves talking to and convincing yourself that you can push through the pain and have a successful workout. Self-coaching, while beneficial in and of itself, also helps you to use relaxation and imagery techniques more effectively.

The Four Stages of Pain

To begin the process of self-coaching, it may be helpful to break down pain into four stages. These four stages are similar to the stages of a workout presented in chapter 6 but on a shorter, more concentrated time frame. The ability to coach yourself through a workout and a painful situation are both

Imagery Practice #1

Using a timer, try each one of the six imagery techniques explained previously for three minutes. Close your eyes during each one, except for external attention diversion. Once you have tried each technique (total time: 18 minutes), answer the following questions.

1. Which two methods did you find the easiest to execute for the full three minutes?

   _____

   _____

2. Which two methods were the most difficult?

   _____

   _____

3. How could these techniques be improved to help you execute them? For example, would being more specific be helpful? If so, make some adjustments before practicing the next time.

   _____

   _____

Imagery Practice #2

Over the next two weeks, try using each of the imagery techniques to control your pain during difficult training sets. After you have been able to try each one at least once, answer the following questions.

1. Which two methods did you find the easiest to execute for the full training set?

   _____

   _____

2. Which two methods were the most difficult?

   _____

   _____

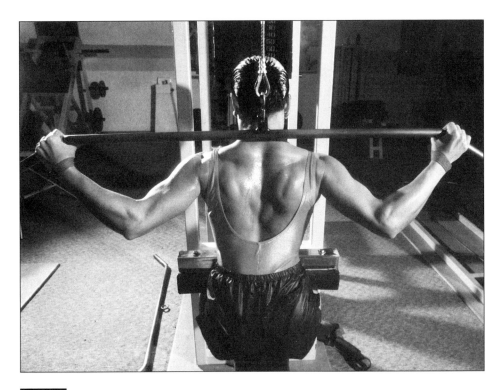

You must mentally prepare yourself before an intense workout.

essential to optimal bodybuilding. Remember, self-coaching involves positive self-talk. Encouraging yourself and staying positive will go a long way toward a successful performance.

Stage 1: Preparation.   Recognize that you are going to experience pain in your workout and begin to prepare for it. Rather than feel overwhelmed and helpless at the onset of pain, develop a coping plan beforehand. This plan could include keeping a positive attitude, stopping negative thoughts as soon as they occur, and redirecting your attention using one of the six imagery techniques explained earlier. Some examples of statements you could use: "Stop worrying about the next painful set; what I can do instead is focus my attention on counting backward from 1,000 by 7" (internal attention diversion), or "I am feeling anxious, but that is natural. There is no reason to decrease intensity at this point. I'll just breathe deeply and relax."

Stage 2: Confrontation.   When you start to feel the pain, use the plan you developed in stage 1, preparation. If necessary, switch strategies and use positive self-talk to coach yourself. For example, you could say: "All right, I'm feeling some pain. That lets me know that the muscle is working. I should take some slow, deep breaths and repeat a cue word that reminds me to keep my mind off the pain. I will repeat the acronym RIMS to remember to *relax*, use *imagery*, and utilize *mental skills* to manage the pain."

Stage 3: Critical Moments. Even if you have a well-developed plan in place to cope with pain during a high-intensity workout, critical moments will likely arise. For example, the pain you experience may surpass what you anticipated and planned for, and you may feel like you need to stop because it hurts too much. When you find yourself giving way to unpleasant thoughts or feelings—"It hurts" or "I have to quit"—make an effort to stop them. Use your self-coaching skills to get back on track. Remember, if the pain is in the belly of the muscle then it is likely a healthy form of pain and you must learn to push through it. Relying on the various imagery techniques, discussed earlier, will go a long way toward getting you through the most intense moments of training. Exercise that leads to joint pain, a good predictor of future injury, should not be continued. It is a wise bodybuilder that learns to push through safe critical moments and stop lifting in situations of potential injury.

Stage 4: Reflection. In the beginning of your pain-management strategy, you may notice only a small change in your ability to tolerate pain. Do not be discouraged. This is a new skill, one that will take practice to perfect. Give yourself a pat on the back for taking even a small step toward pain management. Controlling your pain during high-intensity workouts will bring you that much closer to achieving the toned, sculpted body you desire. If you have managed to control your pain even a little bit, you deserve to feel proud.

Create Practice Opportunities

It is crucial that you experiment with the various breathing, relaxation, and mental skills presented throughout this book. Your personality, life experiences, and athletic background all play a role in determining which methods are best for you. Once you have eliminated the techniques you consider ineffective, select two or three that you want to use. Practice these techniques at home and during every training set, even easy sets. The better you are at using these techniques during easy training sets, the more effective they will become during difficult sets.

In the end, a higher level of pain tolerance will allow you to work out at higher intensities. This will in turn boost your self-confidence, which will enable you to use pain-management techniques in future, and possibly aversive, training scenarios. Exercises 7.3 through 7.5 provide the opportunity to practice and perfect some of your skills. While you are going through the exercises, use the two or three mental skills you are most comfortable with.

Exercise 7.3 | Ice Water Task

Instructions: You will need a timer for this exercise. Place your hand into a bucket of ice water. You will experience some pain, but the pain is not damaging and is instantly relieved by removing your hand from the water. Try holding your hand in the water for one minute, then two minutes, then three minutes, and so on. Replenish the ice and change hands between trials. Practice as much as possible, trying to hold your hand in the water as long as possible. Write any comments or observations in the space provided below.

Trial 1:

Trial 2:

Trial 3:

Trial 4:

Exercise 7.4 | Phantom Chair Task

Instructions: You will need a timer for this exercise. Stand with your back against a wall and slide down the wall until your thighs are parallel with the floor. (This would be the exact same position as sitting in a chair, except that there is no chair below you.) You will feel a pain in your thighs as you try to hold the position. Like the ice water task, try to hold the position for one minute, then two minutes, then three minutes, and so on. After each trial, take at least a 15-minute break. You may want to do only one trial each day. While you are experiencing the pain, try to use some of the mental skills you've acquired to handle it more effectively. Write any comments or observations in the space provided below.

Trial 1:

Trial 2:

Trial 3:

Trial 4:

Exercise 7.5 | Lifting Task

Instructions: Pick two mental skills you feel comfortable with (for example, relaxation response, imagery, or self-coaching) and use them during a difficult training set. Try to use one throughout each set. The more you practice the skill in a training set, the more likely you will be able to use the skill throughout a workout. Write any comments or observations below.

Trial 1:

Trial 2:

Trial 3:

Trial 4:

Mental Toughness

In every sport, athletes and coaches talk about being mentally tough. Indeed, the importance of mental toughness is touted on sports radio and television programs, and in newspapers worldwide. What, exactly, is this elusive quality of mental toughness, and how does a bodybuilder attain it?

In his book *Sports Slump Busting*,[4] Dr. Alan Goldberg explains that mental toughness is a combination of learned skills that help you raise your level of training and competitive performance. He identifies six different skills critical to being mentally tough.

1.   Goal setting. Understanding how to use goals to develop optimal levels of motivation is an important first step in becoming mentally tough. It is important to know the secrets to effective goal setting, discussed in chapter 8, and to know why so many bodybuilders falter in their body-sculpting journey. The mental skills described in this book, including relaxation, imagery, and self-coaching, are invaluable tools in staying focused on your bodybuilding dreams.

2.   Stress management. You will not be able to perform to your potential in the gym, or on the stage, unless you have the ability to stay relaxed and focused. One of the most stressful aspects of competitive bodybuilding is the constant attempt to "psyche out" fellow competitors while they train or show off to the judges. The bodybuilder who is best able to handle stress and use it as a tool for improvement is most likely to succeed. This is best accomplished by using a combination of relaxation, imagery, and mental skills.

3.   Self-confidence. Winners exude confidence and losers exude a fragile self-image. Bodybuilders and fitness champions such as Ronnie Coleman, Flex Wheeler, Vicky Gates, and Mary Yockey know how hard they have worked to get the bodies they have. They know that they are among the best in the world and have an aura of confidence around them. How do you build self-confidence? How do you effectively deal with doubts about your body and the negative thinking that can easily stop you in your tracks? You must learn to coach yourself so that you maintain a winning self-confidence, regardless of who is in the gym or on stage beside you.

4.   Reboundability. Bouncing back from setbacks, losses, and bad breaks is critical to your bodybuilding success. You will face many obstacles on your way to the pinnacle of body development. Learning how to use these obstacles to get closer to your goals is critical. Remember, every bodybuilder faces obstacles. It is the one who is best able to overcome them who rises to the top. Use failure as a learning tool and a guide for future training.

5.   Concentration. Your ability to concentrate and work with intensity is the key to body excellence. It is easy to be distracted by good music, friends, and attractive bodies at the gym, but do not let it happen. Do not let

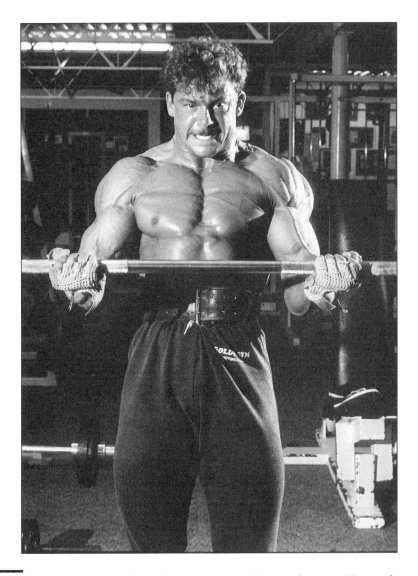

Mental toughness is crucial for enhancing your training and competitive performance.

distractions take you away from your training for more than a moment, and learn to focus on reaching your potential. At the core of mental toughness are concentration skills. Learn to focus on what is important and block out everything else.

6. Imagery and visualization. Successful bodybuilders see how they want to look in their mind's eye, while those who are not successful can only see how they look now. Imagery and visualization are crucial in seeing yourself the way you want to look and knowing it will happen. Moreover, imagery and visualization help you develop confidence, overcome fears, and avoid "psyche outs" and intimidation by other bodybuilders.

Pain tolerance is an important mental skill that can be developed by any bodybuilder. The ability to tolerate intense workouts and push through painful situations will help you overcome the training plateaus that are commonplace in bodybuilding. Anticipating the pain in training and being prepared for it will put you far ahead of your competition. You may even look forward to the pain in training and the results that pushing through it can provide.

CHAPTER 8

Overcoming Inertia and Breaking Through Plateaus

Over the years, you have probably been bombarded with statistics proving the myriad benefits of a physically active life. It may even be the reason you got into bodybuilding. Knowledge about exercise and its benefits is not enough, however. You see, it is estimated that as much as 80 percent of those who join a gym or fitness center will stop going within the first three months. It could be that they get bored, aren't seeing results, or are simply too busy to make exercise a priority. Experienced bodybuilders also experience times when they aren't seeing the changes to their physique they desire. The point is every person engaged in bodybuilding and fitness will have training plateaus or times when they lack motivation.

The challenge for many bodybuilders, including those in the elite category, is learning to push themselves through the training plateaus and sticking with a workout or nutrition regimen. To keep yourself from becoming another statistic, it is important that you understand your motivation for exercise; learn to set goals for your physical training, nutrition planning, and lifestyle patterns; and get a better grasp of time management. In addition to these topics, this chapter also provides guidelines for periodizing your training, reworking your nutrition program, and creating a new mind-set to help you break through the plateaus of training.

Motivation

Personality theorists often talk about an impermeable part of our personality that is largely unaffected by the world around us. The nature of our personality core is revealed to us as we age and begin to learn more about who we are and what makes us tick. It is the same for motivation. Deep within lies a motivational core that influences you to enjoy some activities more than others, to associate with certain types of people, and to act in certain ways. For example, some bodybuilders are so afraid of failing that they are unwilling to stick it out. Others are perfectionists who would prefer not to exercise at all given the chance they will not achieve the perfect body: "If I can't look like Cory Everson, why do it?" Still others are simply underachievers who set their goals far below their abilities.

Understanding your motivation for exercise is the first step in sticking with your program. Your motivational core, which determines the exercise activities you like and dislike, is ultimately at the center of sticking with your program and breaking through plateaus.

You are probably well aware of what motivates you to be a bodybuilder. Perhaps your motivation is a significant person in your life, a psychological fear of being overfat, or a strong desire to be fit and healthy. The problem is, most bodybuilders are aware only of what motivates them, not what de-motivates them. All people have things in their life that suck the energy out of their desire to do something.

Having a good grasp of the forces that affect motivation is crucial to an effective training program. Knowing what de-motivates you enables you to control it. I have known bodybuilders who were motivated to lose 10 pounds of body fat until a spouse or loved one said they would never be able to do it. Unaware of the power others had on their motivation level, these bodybuilders gave up. The motivation they had for losing body fat was weak enough that one offhanded comment brought them down. Simply put, their de-motivation was stronger than their motivation. Use exercise 8.1 to assess your own motivation.

The reality is that unless you are able to break through training plateaus and continue training, you will never reach your bodybuilding goals. In fact, it is far more important to train than it is to know how to train. The best training program is the one you consistently use. Once you are aware of what de-motivates you, it becomes possible to (1) begin to strengthen your motivation so that it is not as susceptible to negative factors, and (2) reduce the effect of de-motivational forces, rendering them unable to steer you off course.

1. Select and rank the reasons you became a bodybuilder.

( ) To improve overall health
( ) To improve fitness to help in daily tasks
( ) To look good in beach attire
( ) Girlfriend/boyfriend/spouse encouraged me
( ) Tired of being skinny
( ) Tired of being overweight
( ) Want to look like the fit people in magazines and on television
( ) To get a girlfriend/boyfriend
( ) To help me through the work day
{ } Enjoy the weight-training process
{ } An opportunity to expand my social circle

Other reasons:

( ) _____
( ) _____
( ) _____

2. Of the reasons you selected for becoming a bodybuilder, rate the motivational influence of the top six. The rating scale ranges from 1 to 10, with 10 indicating the strongest influence.

3. Select and rank those things that you do not like about being a bodybuilder.

( ) Intensity of training
( ) Strict adherence to nutrition regimen
( ) Comparing my body with those of other bodybuilders
( ) Gym environment
( ) Tight and/or skimpy clothing
( ) Pressure to take performance-enhancing substances
( ) Lack of friends in bodybuilding
( ) Lack of girlfriend/boyfriend/spouse in bodybuilding
( ) Financial cost
( ) Muscle soreness and/or injury
( ) Social stigma toward bodybuilding

(continued)

Others:

( ) _____

( ) _____

( ) _____

4. Of the things you do not like about bodybuilding, rate the de-motivational influence of the top six. The rating scale ranges from 1 to 10, with 10 indicating the strongest influence.

5. Total the scores for questions 2 and 4. Then subtract the question 4 total from the question 2 total. Find the difference in the following categories to understand the strength of your motivational core for bodybuilding.

Question 2 total ___

Question 4 total ___

Difference (question 2 total − question 4 total) ___

50 to 60 points: Your motivational core for bodybuilding is excellent. You do not let anything negative get in the way of your goal of becoming as muscular as you can. Your exuberance may cause you to forget that bodybuilding is a hierarchical climb toward body perfection requiring discipline over time, but if you allow yourself to "smell the flowers" you will truly be awesome.

40 to 49 points: You are well suited to the bodybuilding lifestyle. You are positively orientated but also recognize that there are some things in life that can suck away your motivation. Learn to change those things that can negatively affect your motivation level and to accept those things that you cannot change. Reading positive articles in muscle magazines and on the internet will help you to keep positive.

30 to 39 points: You are well suited to the bodybuilding lifestyle but are not sure that you will be able to stick with it. Remember that there will be negative influences in your life and that they will affect your commitment levels. Take control over negative influences and begin by educating yourself more on the positive things that you can do to enhance motivation for bodybuilding.

20 to 29 points: You do have a positive orientation to being a bodybuilder but you are also affected in a big way by negative influences in your life. Take steps to eliminate those negative influences if at all possible. If you cannot eliminate them then you must learn to accept them and allow your positive influences to become better developed. Take time to talk to other serious bodybuilders and personal trainers at your gym to see how you can become more positive in your bodybuilding outlook.

10 to 19 points: You are allowing negative influences to take your heart and mind away from bodybuilding. You do see something positive about the bodybuilding lifestyle but do not see that it is a viable option for you. The negative influences are very strong and if you are going to adhere to bodybuilding you will need to get control of them. Take time to review the positives and negatives that you identified and see if there is any way you can make the positives a stronger influence on your life.

Less than 10 points: You will have to re-evaluate whether bodybuilding is the activity for you. If you still believe that you want to be a bodybuilder then you will have to enhance your positive motivation level. Read some good bodybuilding magazines such as *Muscle and Fitness* and pick up a good self-motivation book from the local bookstore

---

Strategies for Sticking With Your Program and Breaking Through Plateaus

Just as there is more than one personality type among bodybuilders, there are many ways to break through training plateaus. Which strategy you choose will depend on your personality, previous experience with training plateaus, the training environment, and the level of social support you get for bodybuilding. The rest of the chapter outlines a number of different strategies that you may or may not be familiar with. Read through each of them carefully and choose two or three that you want to try the next time you are in a "flat" situation. Figure 8.1 illustrates the relationship between your motivational core and the various strategies for breaking through plateaus.

Strategy #1. Set Individual Goals

Would you try to find your way around a new city without a road map? Probably not. But that is just what athletes do in sport: they continually try to improve their performance without a road map to follow. Bodybuilders are no different.

The best way to strengthen your motivational core for bodybuilding is to set goals and develop strategies to accomplish them. It is particularly important to establish some individual goals and strategies at the start of every year. Setting goals is helpful in two ways: (1) Goal setting will allow you to focus your energy on tasks specific to body improvement; and (2) goals can provide motivation when you review and evaluate them regularly. Goal setting is one of the most important skills you can use to break through training plateaus and prevent future plateaus.

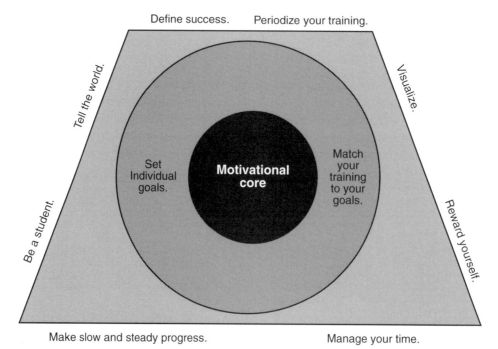

Figure 8.1 Relationship between motivational core and strategies for breaking through plateaus.

The most common goal-setting method among bodybuilders is not very productive. Typically, bodybuilders will determine the type of body they would like, usually as a haphazard exercise, while watching television, eating dinner, or reading a bodybuilding magazine. Half-serious bodybuilders are no better. Many will take the time to think about goals, but they merely write their goals down on a scrap of paper, in the event that they will want to review them at a future time.

There are three major problems with these typical goal-setting scenarios. First, if and when bodybuilders decide to review their goals, they will not be able to remember exactly what they decided because they did not write them down, or they will not be able to find the scrap of paper they wrote them on. After all, why take the time to write down goals if you are unable to review them in a systematic and purposeful way? Second, bodybuilders fail to evaluate their strengths and weaknesses or get others' opinions about the validity of their goals. Perhaps the goals are unrealistic. Third, the most important aspect of goal setting is determining the process for goal achievement. Even though you may not achieve every goal, if you work toward each goal with a systematic plan, you have a good chance of achieving a significant portion of them.

If you remember chapter 1, you will recall that serious bodybuilders should conduct a comprehensive evaluation of their bodybuilding strengths and weaknesses in the areas of muscular development, nutritional habits, lifestyle patterns, and mental skills. In addition to setting goals in these critical areas, it is also wise to set goals in training and performance. You should set goals in the following areas.

• *Performance.* Performance goals consist of short-term, long-term, and dream goals. Short-term goals are those you would like to accomplish in the next four to six weeks, long-term goals are those you would like to reach this year, and dream goals are those you would like to attain in the next two to three years. While goal setting related to outcomes and comparison (for example, winning a competition or beating a particular opponent) is often appropriate to competitive bodybuilders, most bodybuilders find it best to emphasize achievement goals related to individual progress and best personal performance.

• *Muscular-development.* These are goals related to the development of the muscular frame, including the size of various muscle groups, body symmetry, strength, flexibility, and power.

• *Nutrition.* Nutrition goals could include the ways you prepare food and what you ingest, for example, fats, carbohydrates, proteins, nutritional supplements, and sport drinks.

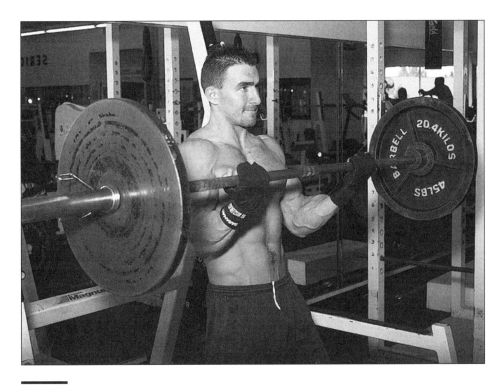

Knowing yourself and recognizing your strengths and weaknesses is the first step toward effective goal-setting.

- *Lifestyle pattern.* Lifestyle pattern goals include those aspects of your lifestyle that may affect body development, including sleeping patterns, the use of recreational drugs and alcohol, social activities, and so on.

- *Mental skills.* As discussed throughout this book, mental skill is critical to any effective training program. Mental skill goals include acquiring any and all tools that enable you to create a positive mind-set, improve your motivation, and gain emotional control, including relaxation, visualization, imagery, concentration, self-coaching, and so on.

- *Training.* Training goals are related to your training program in the gym. For example, how often you train, when you train, and what you would like to accomplish during individual training sessions. Goal setting in the training category may also include commitment to and intensity of training sessions.

- *Behavior.* Goals that focus on the way you think and behave in the gym and on stage are behavior goals. What type of attitude would you like to have toward your training partner, competitors, judges, and spectators? Behavior goals may also include the ways that you want to think and behave while training or during competitions.

Goal-Setting Guidelines

There are many different ways to set goals and, for the most part, they can all be effective, depending on the characteristics and preferences of each individual. Nevertheless, many studies have come up with a number of common factors associated with effective goal setting.

Set Difficult but Realistic Goals.   Research shows that the more difficult the goal, the better the athlete's performance. But this is true only if achieving that goal is realistic. For example, if you are a recreational bodybuilder, it may not be appropriate to set a goal of entering a regional bodybuilding championship by the end of the year. This will only result in frustration and failure.

Set Short-Term, Long-Term, and Dream Goals.   As shown in figure 8.2, goal setting is like climbing a set of stairs. Your ultimate goal may be to reach the top of the stairs, but to do that you must take one small step at a time. Short-term goals are those steps. They provide the motivation to stay on track with your training. By starting with your short-term goals, before you know it, you will have reached your long-term goal. At that point, you will be that much closer to achieving your dream.

While you should set long-term and dream goals, it is essential for you to establish short-term goals. Short-term goals allow you to see immediate improvements in performance and, in doing so, enhance your motivation. Ideally, you should first set a long-term goal (six months to one year) that is realistic, yet challenging. Working backward, set a series of short-term goals (four to six weeks) that will lead to accomplishing your long-term goal.

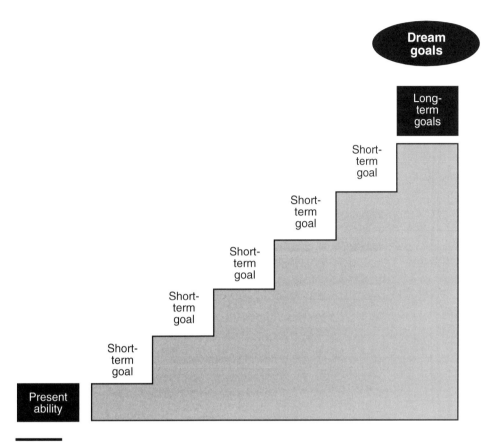

Figure 8.2 Relationship of short-term, long-term, and dream goals.

Finally, building on your long-term goal, set a dream goal (two to three years) that reflects your ultimate vision of success. The following is an example of a proper term-goal progression.

1. Long-term goal:

   "I will increase the size of my upper arms 1 inch by the end of the year."

2. Short-term goals:

   "I will complete 4 sets of barbell curls using the pyramid training technique."

   "I will be sure to keep the intensity high during my tricep training."

   "I will specifically train my biceps and triceps only once per week."

   "I will vary the speed and number of repetitions during each workout to shock my muscles into growth."

   "I will learn as much as I can about arm development in the next two weeks by reading bodybuilding magazines and talking with personal trainers."

3. Dream goal:

"I want to compete at the NPC National Bodybuilding Championships in the next four years."

Set Specific Goals in Measurable Terms. Goals that are specific are more effective in facilitating an effective training program than are general goals, for example, "I will do my best." After finishing a training session, you may find it difficult to determine whether you actually did perform your best or not. To evaluate your progress and measure your success, your goals must be specific and measurable, such as increasing your lifts by a specific amount of weight each session. By using a measurable goal, you will know immediately after each training session whether or not you accomplished your goal.

Set Performance Goals, Not Outcome Goals. As explained earlier in this chapter, it may be easy to set a goal to win a championship or have the largest quadriceps in the gym, but this type of goal, called "outcome goals," is far less effective than performance goals—if for no other reason than the outcome of a competition is largely out of your control. You may perform at your very best yet not win the competition. Your quadriceps may be as big as they have ever been and still not be the biggest in the gym. Moreover, whether or not you are the best or the biggest depends on whom you compare yourself to.

Set Specific Goals for Lifting Weights

This is a formula based on the work of O'Block and Evans.[1] Called "interval goal setting (IGS)," the formula allows you to set weight-lifting goals that are challenging and based on objective criteria—your past lifting scores. This eliminates the guesswork of setting proper goals. Shown below is an example of the IGS model for the last five personal best bench presses by a competitive bodybuilder. The bench press lifts were 330, 320, 340, 345, 350.

A = 337 (average of 5 lifts)

B = 350 (best of 5 lifts)

C = 13 (difference between average and best lift) (350 - 337)

D = 350 (lower interval boundary; performer's best lift out of 5 performances)

E = 363 (interval midpoint) (350 + 13)

F = 376 (upper interval boundary) (363 + 13)

The appropriate goal to set for bench press would be 363-376.

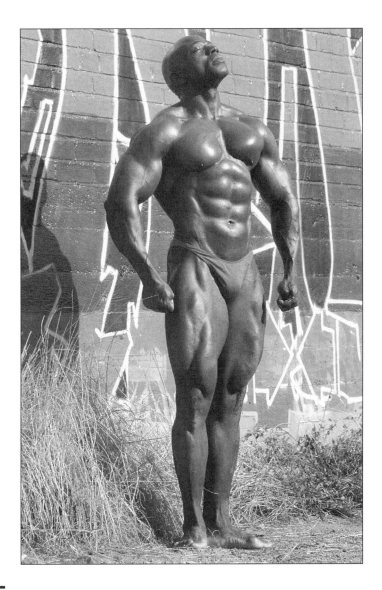

Focusing on achieving success, rather than avoiding failure, is the essence of positive goal setting.

You cannot control your standing among other bodybuilders in the gym, but you can take charge of the way you develop your body. By establishing personal performance goals, you will create better opportunities to achieve your definition of success. You will also learn to judge success and failure in terms of your own body, not on the basis of peer comparison.

Set Positive Goals, Not Negative Goals. Goals can be stated in either positive terms ("I will increase the amount of protein I eat") or negative terms ("I will decrease the number of times I eat high-fat foods"). As much as is possible, state your goals in terms of the way you want to behave, as opposed to the way you do not want to behave. Stating your goals in positive terms will help you focus on what you need to do to accomplish your goal rather than on what you do not need to do. Put another way, positive goal setting focuses on achieving success rather than avoiding failure.

Identify Target Dates. Establishing a target date for goal completion will help motivate you to accomplish your goals sooner rather than later. Allow the time within your target date to evaluate whether you reached your goal. If you succeeded, you will need to set a new goal. If you fell a bit short of your goal, keep your original goal and set a new target date. If you missed your goal altogether, you may need to adjust it so that it is more realistic.

Identify Achievement Strategies. The most important ingredient in goal setting is not the goals themselves but what you plan to do to reach them. Too often goals are established but never achieved because bodybuilders have failed to identify strategies for achieving them. Once you have set your goals, identifying achievement strategies is a two-step process.

1. Create action steps that will help you to reach your goals. For example, let's say that your goal is to increase your bench press by 25 pounds. Action steps will specify exactly what you are going to do to meet that goal. These may include

   - spending workout time focusing on those muscle groups responsible for benching,
   - adjusting your eating regimen to ensure adequate protein for muscle growth,
   - beginning a nutritional supplementation program that includes 5 to 10 grams of creatine or glutamine for muscle growth, and
   - talking to a strength coach twice each month about lifting technique and muscle development.

2. Now that you have set action steps, it is time to identify barriers that may get in the way of achieving your goal. It is important to identify potential barriers and deal with them before they become a problem. Does time on the job take away from adequate time in the gym? Does your spouse or partner want you to stay home rather than go to the gym? Do you have an active social life that encourages poor nutritional habits? Make a plan to deal with these potential barriers so that they will not interfere with reaching your goals. For example, you could arrange a time to exercise that fits with your job situation or discuss your exercise goals with your spouse or partner and find ways to spend quality time together.

Record Your Goals. Too often bodybuilders set goals but then fail to write them down. This is okay in the beginning, because most bodybuilders are motivated enough to remember them in the short term. Over the course of a year-long training program marked by many ups and downs, however, it is common to forget exactly which goals were established. It is both wise and useful to write your goals down and place them in a location where you will be able to refer back to them easily.

Evaluate Your Goals. Periodic evaluation, ideally every six weeks, is absolutely necessary if your goals are to enhance performance. Through evaluation, you will likely find that you have already achieved some of your long-term goals, perhaps because they were too easy, and thus will have to set new long-term goals. Conversely, you may find that some of your long-term goals were too difficult and need to be readjusted. In the evaluation process, it may be useful to get feedback from an outside but knowledgeable source on your short-term and long-term goals.

Setting Your Own Goals

Now that you understand the ins and outs of goal setting, you can use the following pages to set your bodybuilding goals, identify possible barriers to achieving those goals and determine appropriate action steps, and evaluate your goals. As you complete exercises 8.2 through 8.4, keep the following in mind.

- Goal setting can motivate you to prepare and execute your desired performance as well as provide you with direction.
- Set one goal for each training session and then decide after the session whether you met the goal. Make any necessary adjustments.
- The purpose of setting goals is to change your behavior. Do not waste time and energy on things you cannot control. You can only change what you can control.
- You must commit to your goals. Without total commitment to your goals, you will not put in the effort required to meet them.
- You must be aware of your strengths and weaknesses to set challenging but realistic goals. Use the information you gained from the awareness exercises in chapter 1 to set your goals according to your strengths and weaknesses.
- Goals do not come easily. As the year progresses, you will likely experience more pressure as you try to accomplish your goals. Do not stray. Stay focused on your goals and, sooner or later, you will accomplish more than you believe possible.
- Effective goal setting takes practice. The more experience you have setting goals, the more proficient you will become at it.
- Get feedback. Discuss your goals with your spouse, friends, training partner, and significant others to help you set goals that are as realistic as possible.

Exercise 8.2 | Individual Goal-Setting Sheet

Name _____ Date _____ Target date _____

PERFORMANCE GOALS

Instructions: List your short- and long-term goals for the next year and dream goals for the next 2-3 years (these may include an emphasis on the outcome of a competition such as, winning a competition or beating a particular opponent), emphasizing achievement goals that are related to achieving your best personal performance. Achievement-orientated performance goals reflect an increased perceived ability, mastery of new tasks, or skill improvement. This is in contrast to performance goals that are more concerned with the process and not the final product.

Short-term goals:

Long-term goals:

Dream goals:

MUSCULAR DEVELOPMENT GOALS

Instructions: List goals related to the development of your muscular frame, including body symmetry, strength, flexibility, power, and the size of various muscle groups.

NUTRITIONAL HABITS GOALS

Instructions: List your nutrition goals, including what you eat and how you prepare food. These can include eating fats, carbohydrates, and proteins; taking supplements; consuming sport drinks; and cooking nutritious meals.

LIFESTYLE PATTERNS GOALS

Instructions: List goals that relate to aspects of your lifestyle that may affect body development. These can include, sleeping patterns, use of recreational drugs and alcohol, and social activities.

(continued)

MENTAL SKILL GOALS

Instructions: List goals for achieving the mental skills necessary for peak performance. These can include such things as, relaxation, visualization, concentration, and self-coaching.

TRAINING GOALS

Instructions: List goals that refer to how you train in the gym. This may include how often you train, when you train, and what you would like to accomplish during training sessions. You may also want to include goals about commitment and the intensity of training sessions.

BEHAVIORAL GOALS

Instructions: List goals that focus on the way you think and behave in the gym and on stage. What type of attitude would you like to have toward your training partner, competitors, judges, and spectators? You may want to include goals for mentally preparing for training, shows, and competitions.

Exercise 8.3 | Barriers and Action Steps to Goals

PERFORMANCE GOALS

Carefully think about those things that might prevent you from achieving your goals. Becoming aware of them will help you overcome them. After you have determined the barriers, list detailed action steps. Action steps are specific plans to reach your goals.

Action steps: Put into sequence the action steps necessary to achieve your goals.

Short-term goals

1.

2.

3.

4.

5.

Long-term goals

1.

2.

3.

4.

Dream goals

1.

2.

3.

Barriers: List obstacles that may prevent you from achieving your goals. How will you deal with these obstacles?

1.

2.

3.

(continued)

MUSCULAR DEVELOPMENT GOALS

Action steps: Put into sequence the action steps necessary to achieve your goals.

1.

2.

3.

4.

Barriers: List obstacles that may prevent you from achieving your goals. How will you deal with these obstacles?

1.

2.

NUTRITIONAL HABIT GOALS

Action steps: Put into sequence the action steps necessary to achieve your goals.

1.

2.

3.

4.

Barriers: List obstacles that may prevent you from achieving your goals. How will you deal with these obstacles?

1.

2.

LIFESTYLE PATTERNS GOALS

Action steps: Put into sequence the action steps necessary to achieve your goals.

1.

2.

3.

4.

Barriers: List obstacles that may prevent you from achieving your goals. How will you deal with these obstacles?

1.

2.

MENTAL SKILLS GOALS

Action steps: Put into sequence the action steps necessary to achieve your goals.

1.

2.

3.

4.

Barriers: List obstacles that may prevent you from achieving your goals. How will you deal with these obstacles?

1.

2.

TRAINING GOALS

Action steps: Put into sequence the action steps necessary to achieve your goals.

1.

2.

3.

4.

Barriers: List obstacles that may prevent you from achieving your goals. How will you deal with these obstacles?

1.

2.

BEHAVIORAL GOALS

Action steps: Put into sequence the action steps necessary to achieve your goals.

1.

2.

3.

4.

Barriers: List obstacles that may prevent you from achieving your goals. How will you deal with these obstacles?

1.

2.

Exercise 8.4 | Goal Achievement Card

Instructions: Pick one muscle group that you would like to evaluate. Choose three exercises for that muscle group. Rate yourself on each exercise. Then set a specific goal, strategy, and target date for achievement.

Name_____ **Date**_____

Muscle group_____ **Training stage/goal**_____

Exercise	Rating			Specific goal	Strategy	Target date
	Strong	Average	Poor			

Strategy #2. Match Your Training to Your Goals

The second strategy for breaking through training plateaus is to ensure your training program will actually help you meet your goals. How long would you stick with a program that was not giving you any noticeable results? I once counseled a girl who was frustrated with her exercise program. She wanted to tone up but after four months had not seen any results. She told me that she was on an anaerobic interval-running program three times per week. Wrong program! Her goal was to look better in a swimsuit, not to win a spot on the Olympic track team. She needed a program consisting of weight training, aerobic exercise, and appropriate nutrition.

Inappropriate programs lead to nonadherence. This is why beginners should seek the assistance of certified fitness trainers. A trainer can design the best program for your goals and individual needs. Following a program uniquely designed for you will not only be more effective for achieving your goals, but it will provide measurable, intermediate goals to evaluate your progress against. Moreover, a personal trainer is someone you can be accountable to.

Strategy #3. Be a Student

Elite athletes live and breathe their sport. They spend endless hours playing, watching, and learning about it. You may not need this level of dedication to succeed in bodybuilding, but there is a lesson to be learned. The more you know about bodybuilding, the more likely you will stick with it. Knowledge enhances motivation, which leads to deeper levels of commitment.

Read as much as you can about weight training, bodybuilding, nutrition, and aerobic exercise. Attend fitness seminars and clinics put on by exercise specialists. Search the internet for bodybuilding sites that provide valuable information to novice and advanced bodybuilders. Pick up a fitness or bodybuilding magazine.

Stretegy #4. Tell the World!

Why are bodybuilders so afraid to tell people their desire to gain 30 pounds of muscle, to look good in a bathing suit, or to have chiseled abdominals? Sure, some bodybuilders go around telling everyone how strong they are or how beautiful they intend to make their bodies, but this is not the norm. Most bodybuilders keep quiet about their bodybuilding goals for fear of being rejected or ridiculed. This is a problem. While I do not suggest that you stick a picture of your head on a professional bodybuilder's body and place it in your back car window for everyone to see, I do suggest that you share your bodybuilding dreams with those who are close to you so that they can help you accomplish your goals.

Research shows that social support plays a powerful role in goal accomplishment and pushing through training plateaus. Something as simple as a verbal reminder or companionship during workouts can really help. Research also shows that weight loss combined with social support and team nutrition programs are far more effective than individual programs. Such support for your training and nutritional programs can come from anyone you consider a significant presence in your life: those who are important to you, those whose opinions you desire, value, and respect. These people may include spouses, parents, peers, children, employers, teachers, friends, counselors, and others.

It is also interesting to note that social support is far more effective for bodybuilders when significant others understand the appropriate eating and exercise patterns involved. In other words, if you do not inform your support network about the hows and whys of your training program, how can you expect them to be supportive of and helpful in accomplishing your goals? Don't be shy! Tell the people in your life about your fitness goals. They will probably be more than willing to help you in your pursuits, and maybe your enthusiasm will get them off the couch!

Strategy #5. Define Success

It is so easy for all of us to fall into the trap of accepting others' values and ideals. Don't get me wrong. Many of these values may be worth adopting, but you still need to decide for yourself. The same goes for how you define *success*. While some bodybuilders may consider themselves successful only if they lift 350 pounds on the bench press or develop 20-inch arms, those goals may not be appropriate for you. Determine your own definition of *success*, and be prepared to celebrate when you reach it. People who experience little successes along the way are more motivated to continue with their bodybuilding program than those who are never satisfied.

Strategy #6. Use Visualization

Visualization can help you in two significant ways: it can improve your workout performance and enhance your motivation. Visualization gives you the power to create your own reality through thoughts, images, and feelings. By envisioning your desired body shape, you will increase the possibility of realizing that vision. Visualization allows you to take control of your fitness potential by giving you a mental image of what and who you can be. Visualizing yourself executing your favorite exercise with strength, power, and flawless execution gives you an energizing sense of confidence. Visualizing the body you want motivates you to stick with the exercise and nutritional program that will ultimately take you there.

While some athletes take longer than others, given enough time and practice, almost everyone is able to visualize. Terry Orlick, in his book *Psyching for Sport*, offers a step-by-step procedure for training athletes to visualize.[2] Use the following sample exercise, adapted from that procedure, to test your visualization skills.

1. Sit down and relax.
2. With your eyes closed, visualize the gym where you train and the equipment you use.
3. Visualize yourself doing a simple, compound exercise.
4. Try to feel the strain or pain of that exercise.
5. Once you are able to do this, try to visualize yourself executing a more complex exercise.

(Hint: Make your visualization as vivid as possible by focusing on physical characteristics and sensations, such as the feel of the equipment surface, the texture of your clothing, the exact colors of your surroundings. The more detailed the images, the more effective the visualization.)

6. Repeat two to three sets of each exercise in your mind, then move on to the next exercise in your routine.

If you have trouble with this procedure, it may be easier to start with a simpler visualization.

1. Hold your hand in front of your face and memorize its detail.
2. Now close your eyes and try to visualize your hand in your mind. (Peeking is allowed until you are able to construct a vivid image in your mind.)
3. Now watch someone executing a weightlifting set and memorize his or her movements.
4. Close your eyes and try to re-create those movements in your mind.

It may also be easier to learn visualization if you are guided through the process. With practice, you will eventually enjoy the process and be able to visualize on your own. The following guidelines, offered in *Sporting Body Sporting Mind*, will help you learn the visualization process.[3]

1. Start with relaxation. Learning a new exercise or executing a familiar exercise is enhanced when you are in a state of relaxed awareness. It is no different with visualization. It is important that physical tension be released so that it will not interfere with the mind-body connection. Use breathing techniques or Benson's Relaxation Response (discussed in chapter 10) for at least five minutes before starting a visualization.

2. Stay alert. Effective visualization requires both relaxation and concentration. Concentration allows for stronger signals, thus creating a clearer image. Begin by visualizing for three minutes. (No visualization session should ever last longer than 10 minutes.) If you notice that your concentration is beginning to waver, end the session and make sure that the next session is shorter.

3. Use present tense. Visualizing in the present makes the images more real and vivid. In other words, when you visualize, imagine that you are performing the exercise right now. Feel your body pushing hard against the weight, experience the emotions, and analyze the mental thought processes you go through as you complete the final reps of a difficult set.

4. Use realistic images. Visualization should correspond directly with the goals you have set. While it is fun to imagine that you are Mr. or Ms. Olympia or that you have just won a competition, it is rarely an effective

strategy. In most cases, it is best to visualize executing a difficult, yet realistic set or competing at a level that is possible with hard work and dedication. As your body becomes more symmetrical and muscular, your visualization can also become more challenging and complex.

5.   Use all your senses. Ideally, visualization should include the visual, auditory, and kinesthetic senses. But many bodybuilders are able to visualize using only their sight. Other bodybuilders find sight difficult and instead stimulate the auditory sense. Everyone is different. To be effective, visualization routines must cater to the individual needs of the bodybuilder. Try the exercise below, adapted from *Sporting Body Sporting Mind,* to help you figure out which of the senses you best respond to.[4]

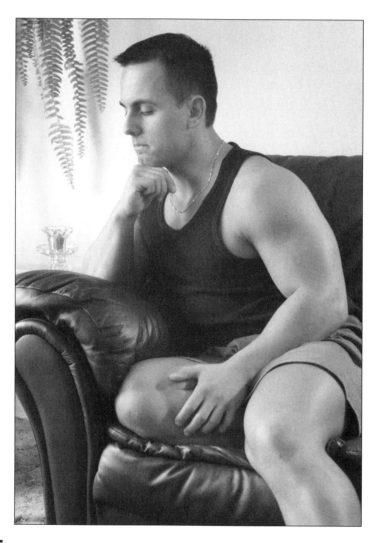

A great way to spend time alone is to practice visualization exercise.

1. Sit comfortably and close your eyes.
2. Take a moment to relax. Breathe deeply.
3. Let yourself imagine, one after another, the following sensory experiences.
   - Imagine a sunset over the ocean . . . an airplane in the sky . . . your favorite piece of workout equipment . . . a famous bodybuilder . . . the face of a relative . . . your favorite room in your house. . . a snow-covered tree . . . a rose as it opens and blooms.
   - Imagine the sound of a rainstorm on a tin roof . . . church bells ringing in the distance . . . the roar of a crowd after the home team has scored the winning point . . . the sound of wind in the trees . . . a favorite piece of music . . . the voice of your training partner . . . the sound of a dog barking.
   - Imagine the feeling of the sun's heat on your back in the afternoon . . . jumping into a hot bath or shower . . . jumping into a cold bath or shower . . . tightening the laces of your sport shoes on each foot . . . the clench of a firm handshake . . . running over a grassy field . . . the pressure of the weight on your arms while doing a bench press.
   - Imagine the smell of burning leaves . . . the smell of the locker room at your gym . . . the smell of bacon frying on the stove . . . the smell of a new piece of equipment or clothing . . . the smell of an indoor swimming pool.
   - Imagine the taste of the bacon you just cooked . . . the taste of a fresh piece of fruit . . . the taste of a protein shake . . . the taste of your favorite food . . . the salty taste of sweat . . . the taste of a cool, refreshing drink after physical exercise.
6. Practice regularly. If possible, practice visualization at the same time and for the same length of time each day. Include visualization as part of your pre-workout routine or at the start of each set. If you are going to make visualization effective, you will need to include it in your overall training program. It is better to practice visualization for three minutes, five days a week, than once a week for 15 minutes. You may feel uncomfortable with the procedure at first, but soon you will enjoy the process and begin to realize its potential in your preparation. If you get bored or frustrated with the same visualization day in and day out, change it. For example, focus on a different aspect of the workout or use background music to make it more exciting.

Content of a Visualization

Visualization starts at the beginning of a training session, competition, or individual exercise. For visualization to be effective, you must know what you want to accomplish and what results you are aiming for. It is often a good idea to watch other successful bodybuilders execute the exercise you are about to do. That way, you get a strong mental picture of exactly how the exercise should be executed, not to mention the image of a bodybuilder performing the motion with strength and power. It is also possible to stimulate effective visualization by drawing each exercise on paper. Draw pictures, cut out photos from magazines, or use descriptive music to help you create a more vivid image.

For example, imagine yourself about to enter the gym, getting ready to work out. In your mind's eye, walk through a typical workout, seeing yourself perform each exercise with flow and perfection. If you see yourself performing an exercise poorly, go back and visualize that exercise again until you perform it with perfection. Use simple focus words such as *strong, relaxed, confident, smooth,* or *centered* as you guide yourself through the entire training session. Become aware of what it feels like to be successful and all the emotions that go along with it. When you are finished with your visualization, bring your attention back to your breathing and slowly begin to reorient yourself to your current surroundings.

Creating Your Own Visualization

If you would prefer, you can create your own visualization. Kay Porter and Judy Foster, in their book *The Mental Athlete,* provide some excellent tips that can be used to create personal visualization for bodybuilding.[5]

- Begin with your arrival at the gym, going through your warm-up routine, and the few minutes before you start training.

- Go into vivid detail about each set and your experience of each exercise, including the sights and sounds in the gym, the color of your clothing and appearance of those around you, the temperature, and the overall atmosphere.

- Imagine yourself totally relaxed, confident, and in complete control of your body and mental state. Feel your confidence, competence, and control. Use affirmations and focus words to help you.

- Go through an entire workout, seeing, feeling, and hearing yourself at each significant point. Feel yourself moving smoothly through each exercise with strength and endurance, in total harmony with the environment and your body.

- After you finish visualizing, jot down some relaxing statements that you can use to remind yourself of your confidence, fitness level, and mental toughness. Tell yourself, "I am a winner."

- Write everything out in the script, then reread and edit what you have written. Once you are satisfied with it, dictate your visualization into your recorder, reading slowly.

- Listen to the tape and make changes to your script. When satisfied, add a progressive relaxation or Relaxation Response message either before or after your visualization. Progressive relaxation and the Relaxation Response will be discussed in chapter 10.

- Listen to the finished tape as often as you wish (Porter and Foster suggest at least once a day) before a training session. Listen to it in your vehicle on the way to the gym. Pick a quiet time and place where you will not be disturbed. In the evening or when you wake up are usually very good times.

A sample of this visualization procedure follows. Record it with music as it is written, or manipulate it to fit your individual needs.

Begin to think of a time in a gym. . . . Remember the confidence and power you felt in the past . . . when your lifting flowed . . . with intensity and focus . . . pushing hard and feeling relaxed and aware in your body. . . . Remember that feeling of control and confidence . . . of being on top of your workouts. . . . See and imagine yourself having the sculptured body you will have. . . being everything you can be . . . everything you are . . . knowing you belong . . . feeling good about how you look and what you are doing . . . knowing deep down inside that you deserve to be in this gym. . . that you are an outstanding bodybuilder. . . . Feel yourself looking, lifting, and feeling confident . . . calm and comfortable with being watched. . . . You are proud, powerful, and in control.

Imagine yourself performing your favorite exercise . . . finishing the way you want to . . . in good form. . . . You are focused and centered on the task . . . paying attention to the mechanics of the lift . . . You know what is happening all the time. . . . You are aware and alert . . . ready for the inevitable intensity. . . . Music is in the background. . . . It invigorates you. . . . You take energy from it . . . always focused on the action and execution. . . . You are enjoying yourself immensely. . . . If you lose your focus, you quickly work to regain it . . . putting your attention and concentration back on the set . . . letting go easily and looking ahead.

You are powerful and strong, and you look forward to the intense discomfort. . . . You know it is about mind over body. . . . You are consistent in your lifting . . . executing each rep and set with passion . . . seeing the blood fill your muscles. . . . You are pushing and pulling like a powerful motor . . . you have a great physique. . . . When you start the next set, you take your time. . . . You relax and lift with intensity and focus . . . keeping your eyes narrowed on the working muscles . . . with power and control.

Feel all those feelings of power, confidence, and control surge through your body . . . lifting hard and intensely . . . with a certain relaxation of mind and body . . . flowing with the set . . . thinking of a word to represent your state of mind. . . . You say the word to yourself . . . eliciting those feelings of power, strength, and muscular pump . . . remembering that your word connects you with that state of mind. . . . Excellence and peak performance . . . feel it in your mind and body. . . . You have what you need to complete this set.

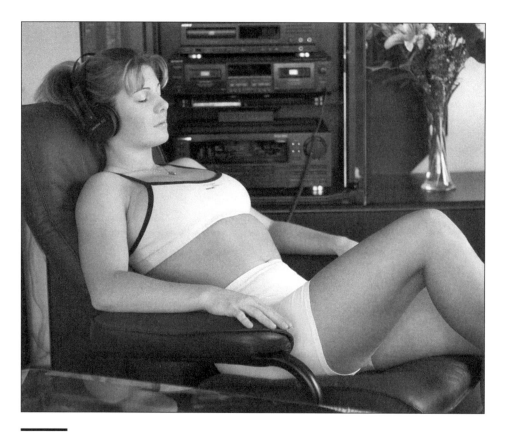

Record your visualization on a tape recorder and listen to the tape before a training session or competition.

Now, slowly let the images fade . . . and become aware of your body sitting or lying down. . . . Know that with every minute of the workout, you are going to get stronger and stronger . . . and more confident. . . . You are now feeling relaxed, refreshed, and ready for the workout . . . ready to go out and lift. . . . Move your hands and feet . . . . Take a deep breath, and let it out with a sigh. . . . Move your neck and shoulders . . . stretch out your legs and arms. . . . Open your eyes and know that you are ready to perform at your best.

Strategy #7. Reward Yourself

Everyone likes to receive gifts, certainly. Why not give yourself a gift for sticking with your program? Treat yourself to a new outfit, a full-body massage, or a weekend holiday. I suggest that all beginners reward themselves at least once per month, regardless of results.

Regardless of results? Are you kidding? No, I am not kidding. I have seen people become frustrated far too often after setting a difficult goal, such as losing 25 pounds.

The problem is not the goal, of course. The problem is that if they wait until they have lost the entire 25 pounds before rewarding themselves, it is likely that they will lose motivation. Not only is this unhelpful, but it can be dangerous. After all, the important thing is not the weight loss but the development of a healthy lifestyle, including exercising regularly and eating sensibly. Thus, if you want to stay motivated, reward yourself for taking steps toward accomplishing your goal—in this case, for making lifestyle changes that will promote fat loss and muscle development. The weight loss will take care of itself.

Strategy #8. Take It Slow and Steady

You have probably heard the story of the tortoise and the hare. The hare started out quickly but was overconfident and decided to rest along the way. Each time the hare rested, the tortoise passed him, eventually winning the race. Think of your bodybuilding program as the race and you as the tortoise. Bodybuilding is not about instant success or quick changes to your body shape; it is about your commitment to a healthy lifestyle of exercise and sound nutrition.

Do not become discouraged when you look at the professional bodybuilders in magazines and at competitions. Most elite bodybuilders have been committed to the bodybuilding lifestyle for many years. (Having the right genetics is a real bonus too.) You will make significant changes in your body shape if you are willing to stick with it. If you keep a log of your workouts and body measurements, when you look back over your progress over the years, you will see that you indeed have won the race.

Strategy #9. Periodize Your Training

Month after month, week after week, day after day, bodybuilders follow the same training and nutrition regimens. Without hesitation, they work their chest and biceps on Mondays, back and triceps on Wednesdays, and legs and shoulders on Fridays. No matter the result, they remain committed, almost like robots, to the same program. It is as if they believe that their muscles will shrink if they change their routine. Nothing could be farther from the truth. In fact, continually doing the same workouts over and over again will lead to stagnation and plateaus in muscle growth.

You must constantly confuse your muscles with different exercises, a combination of different reps and sets, shorter and longer workouts, and easy and difficult sessions. Besides the effect of confusing your muscles, the psychological break you get by varying your training should not be underestimated. Mental breaks lead to a renewed passion and a willingness to do whatever it takes to achieve your very best.

The best way to cycle training, a common process in sport called "periodization," is to divide the training year into one or more periods. Each

The Peaks, Valleys, and Flats of Training: Michael Bodner

Michael Bodner, MSc, CSCS, is the fitness coordinator at the Cambie Community Centre in Richmond, British Columbia. An athlete, trainer, and university educator, Michael's involvement in the fitness industry spans 11 years. Here are some of his thoughts about training plateaus:

Sometimes during the course of training, athletes encounter times when results are greatly reduced or nonexistent. These periods of stagnation are frustrating. This happened to me during my years as a national-class cyclist from time to time, even though I was consistent in my training.

Every time clients or athletes approach me about breaking through their strength or fitness plateaus, I usually begin by investigating their workout history. This means looking not only at their workout from the previous week but also their workout progressions over the past several months. We learn a lot about ourselves from history, and strength-training history is no different. This is why keeping an accurate exercise log is absolutely critical for the serious bodybuilder or athlete.

Including your observations and comments in this log is a good idea. Keeping track of your eating habits or sleeping patterns can reveal that you have not been entirely faithful to your body during the all-important rest phases that encourage muscle growth. Certainly such hidden factors as stress or, possibly, infection can inhibit performance or growth. If these factors can be ruled out, maybe the exercise program itself needs adjustment.

Generally, the temptation is to work harder to overcome the stagnant feeling associated with plateaus. Sometimes the problem is not work intensity but the rest factor. Depending on the type of training program, this may mean more—or less!—rest between sets and workouts. If the lifting intensity is not high enough, I offer my clients some techniques to increase it. For example, I suggest an entire change in the routine if the client has been on the same program for a long time. Assessing the lifting technique itself can also be helpful.

Getting beyond strength or fitness barriers often requires a logical approach. While it is the responsibility of the athlete in question to keep good training records, advice from a trained fitness professional can help make the process more objective.

of these training periods has a unique training focus. The purpose of periodization is to prevent overtraining and optimize peak performance. Periods are usually built around the dates of major competitions. For example, if you are planning to compete in October, you would periodize your training so that you peak at that time.

Why not try to be at your best all the time? That would be impossible. You simply cannot maintain the same muscular size and definition throughout the entire year. There will be times when you need to focus on increasing muscle strength and size and not concern yourself too much with maintaining a ripped physique. It is extremely difficult to gain muscle strength and size while maintaining competitive levels of body fat. So why put yourself under such pressure? Of course, remember the 6 percent rule: no more than 6 percent of your total body weight should be excess body fat during the off-season.

A periodized training plan should include the development of all training factors—muscular size, strength, power, and nutrition—that need to be considered in each of the four bodybuilding periods: muscle building, cutting up, presentation, and transition. For bodybuilders, the muscle-building period can last as long as 36 weeks and has as its primary goal the development of muscle strength and size. The longest, most intense training period, the muscle-building period, contains four distinct phases: hypertrophy/endurance, strength, power, and hypertrophy. Table 8.1 shows the training requirements of muscle building.

The cutting-up period, a difficult period in training, has as its primary goal losing excess body fat while maintaining the muscle earned during the muscle-building period. The biggest change from the muscle-building period to the cutting-up period is the severe adjustment in diet, since diet plays the biggest role in developing a ripped musculature. It is during the six- to eight-week cutting-up period that mental stress is at its highest level. Indeed, it is during the cutting-up period that you may wonder why you became a bodybuilder in the first place. This is when motivation and positive self-talk become critical, because the rewards of your hard work are just around the corner, when your hard-earned muscle will finally be revealed for all to see. Training during the cutting-up period is characterized by high volume (3 to 5 sets of 10 to 15 reps, 16 to 20 sets per workout, 3 to 4 weight-training sessions per week) and low intensity (60 to 70 percent of 1 repetition maximum [RM] with aerobic conditioning (four to five, 30- to 45-minute sessions per week) to encourage loss of body fat.

The presentation period is when you must look your very best, whether that be for a competition, professional appearances, or just showing off your hard-earned physique. To ensure that various muscle groups appear as hard and full as possible, professional bodybuilders time their training and nutrition regimen so that major competitions will fall in the later part of the presentation period. For those of you who have chosen not to compete, it may be best to time the presentation period so that it falls in the summer months when you can show off your body with tank tops, shorts, and bathing suits. Training during this six- to eight-week period should consist of shorter, high-intensity workouts (2 to 4 sets of 8 to 12 reps, 12 to 16 sets per workout, four workouts per week, 65 to 80 percent of 1RM).

Transition is a period of mental and physical rebuilding. It is a time when you can develop other areas of your life. For example, try a new sport, read some books, or go for nice, long walks. Bodybuilding is an intense sport. Thus it is critical that you allow your body and mind to completely break

Table 8.1 Phases of the Muscle-Building Period

PHASE I: HYPERTROPHY

- Training intensity: Low (50-75% of 1RM)
- Training volume: High (3-5 sets of 8-12 reps per exercise)
- Set volume: 18-24 sets per workout
- Rest interval: 60-90 seconds between sets
- Frequency: 4-5 workouts per week
- Length of time: 12-14 weeks

PHASE II: STRENGTH

- Training intensity: High (80-88% of 1RM)
- Training volume: Moderate (3-5 sets of 5-6 reps per exercise)
- Set volume: 14-18 sets per workout
- Rest interval: 90-150 seconds between sets
- Frequency: 3-4 workouts per week
- Length of time: 5-7 weeks

PHASE III: POWER

- Training intensity: Very high (90-95% of 1RM)
- Training volume: Low (3-5 sets of 2-4 reps per exercise)
- Set volume: 12-14 sets per workout
- Rest interval: 150-210 seconds between sets
- Frequency: 3-4 workouts per week
- Length of time: 3-5 weeks

PHASE IV: HYPERTROPHY

- Training intensity: Low (50-75% of 1RM)
- Training volume: High (3-5 sets of 8-12 reps per exercise)
- Set volume: 18-24 sets per workout
- Rest interval: 60-90 seconds between sets
- Frequency: 4-5 workouts per week
- Length of time: 12-14 weeks

Adapted from Wathen 2000.[6]

away from the continual drive for physical perfection. During the four- to six-week transition period, weight training should be reduced to no more than two, 30-minute, full-body workouts per week, and could probably be cut out altogether. When you return to training after the transition period, you will be ready to lift with the renewed passion and intensity necessary for muscle growth.

Periodizing should be thought of not as a restrictive plan but rather as a guide, including enough flexibility to allow for necessary adjustments. Annual periodization becomes a key tool in accomplishing bodybuilding goals, certainly, but it is also a visual reminder of what should happen when.

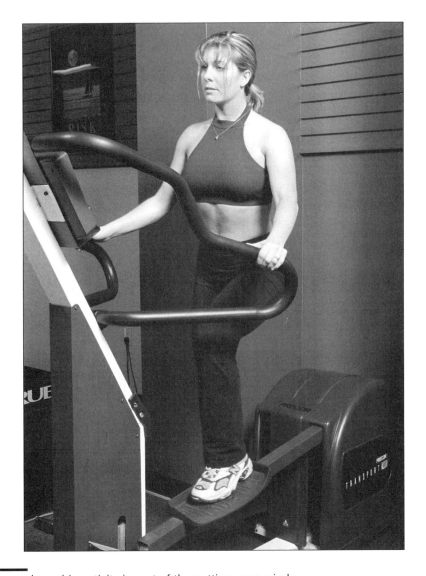

Increased aerobic activity is part of the cutting-up period.

Figure 8.3 is an example of an annual periodized training plan. Depending on your goals, years of bodybuilding experience, and whether you compete, your plan may look quite different.

Strategy #10. Manage Your Time

Have you ever experienced a time lock, when the demands on your time become so overwhelming that it feels impossible to wring one more second out of your already overcrowded schedule? If you have, you are not alone. Research has indicated that nearly 8 out of 10 Americans believe that time moves too quickly, particularly younger adults.

One of the most common reasons that people give for quitting exercise and not pushing through training plateaus is that they are too busy. In this day and age, time has become more valuable than gold for many people. Part of the problem is the myriad roles adults have to play. Females may simultaneously play the roles of girlfriend or wife, mother or grandmother, employee or employer, family social coordinator and budget director, chef, maid, and household manager. Males also must wear a variety of hats simultaneously. Given the amount of time each role requires, it is little wonder that fitness often falls to the wayside.

As a bodybuilder, you know that you must have a sufficient number of training sessions during the week, eat and prepare healthy meals every day, and get a good night's sleep every night to be successful. But is this possible? You bet it is, but you will need to be able to manage your time effectively. The better you manage your time, the less likely that you will be able to use "a lack of time" as an excuse for not exercising.

In many respects, time is similar to money: you have 24 hours to spend each day. You can choose to save ahead (do tasks now so that you will not need to do them later) or spend as you go and borrow from the future (have fun now and hope you find the time to meet your goals later). While the amount of time you have each day remains constant (24 hours), the better you are at time management, the better your chances of achieving the goals you have set for body development. Before you read over the following time-management tips, ask yourself these questions:

- Do I like to procrastinate? Why?
- Do I focus my time on things that are easy or those that must be done?
- How much time am I really using effectively?
- Do I get things done on time? Are they done to my satisfaction?
- Am I comfortable with the pace of my life, or do I feel rushed?
- What sort of planning do I use to manage my time?
- What are my priorities?
- Have I ever weighed the importance of bodybuilding against other aspects of my life?

Training Periods for Advanced Bodybuilders

Name: John Doe

Year: 2000-2001

Months	Oct					Nov				Dec					Jan				Feb				Mar			
Weeks	1	8	15	22	29	5	12	19	26	3	10	17	24	31	7	14	21	28	4	11	18	25	4	11	18	25
Training period	Muscle building																									
Goal	Hypertrophy														Strength				Power				Hyper-trophy			
Type of training	4-5 weight workouts per week 18-24 sets per workout 3-5 sets per exercise 8-12 reps per set 50-75% of 1RM 60-90 seconds rest between sets 20-30 minutes aerobic training 2-3 times per week														3-4 weight workouts per week 14-18 sets per workout 3-5 sets per exercise 5-6 reps per set 80-88% of 1RM 90-150 seconds rest between sets 15-20 minutes aerobic training 2-3 times per week				3-4 weight workouts per week 12-14 sets per workout 3-5 sets per exercise 2-4 reps per set 150-210 seconds rest between sets 15-20 minutes of aerobic training 2-3 times per week				4-5 weight workouts per week 18-24 sets per workout 3-5 sets per exercise 8-12 reps per set 50-75% of 1RM 60-90 seconds rest between sets 20-30 minutes aerobic training 2-3 times per week			

Months	Apr					May				Jun				Jul					Aug				Sep			
Weeks	1	8	15	22	29	6	13	20	27	3	10	17	24	1	8	15	22	29	5	12	19	26	2	9	16	23
Training period	Muscle building									Cutting up				Presentation									Transition			
Goals	Hypertrophy									Fat loss and muscle maintenance				Optimal looks and competition									Recuperation and renewal			
Type of training	4-5 weight workouts per week 18-24 sets per workout 3-5 sets per exercise 8-12 reps per set 50-75% of 1RM 60-90 seconds rest between sets 20-30 minutes aerobic training 2-3 times per week									3-4 weight workouts per week 16-20 sets per workout 3-5 sets per exercise 10-15 reps per set 60-70% of 1RM 45-75 seconds rest between sets 30-45 minutes aerobic training 4-5 times per week				4 weight workouts per week 12-16 sets per workout 2-4 sets per exercise 8-12 reps per set 65-80% of 1RM 60-90 seconds rest between sets 30-45 minutes aerobic training 4-5 times per week									No more than two full-body workouts per week 30-minute workouts Invest time in other activities such as hiking, swimming, cycling, and tennis			

Adapted from Wathan 2000.[7]

Figure 8.3 One-year periodization schedule.

- Would I skip a workout to complete an important work assignment, or vice versa?
- Can the demands of being a bodybuilder and other life roles coexist?

The following time-management tips will help you prioritize your tasks and reduce your stress as you juggle the roles of life and being a bodybuilder.

Avoid Interruptions

When you have a project that requires your full concentration, schedule uninterrupted time. Let your answering machine answer your calls, close your door and put up a "do not disturb" sign, or go to a quiet room where no one will find you. It is so easy to let interruptions take valuable time away from other responsibilities. When you allow yourself to be interrupted, however, you are forced to choose between completing the project now or doing it later and sacrificing something else.

Prioritize Tasks

It is human nature to want to work on the things we most enjoy and not necessarily on those things that are most important. Make a "to do" list for the next day just before going to bed and try to stick to it. Categorize the things you must do that day, the things that need to get done but not immediately, and the things that merely would be nice to get done. When you wake up in the morning, tackle the most important things first. Then work on the tasks that need to get done but not immediately.

Serious bodybuilders love to spend time training in the gym and will often sacrifice other important tasks. The challenge comes when those important tasks have piled up to the point that they are critical. Missing deadlines, performing poorly at work, not completing projects, and missing out on quality time with friends and family make for a very stressful life.

Believe it or not, you can accomplish what you need to in life and still have plenty of time for effective bodybuilding. I recommend scheduling work-outs as a regular part of the weekly schedule. Think of it as scheduling an important meeting with yourself three to four times per week. Treat your bodybuilding with respect. Recognize that if you do not think it is important, no one else will either. Almost nothing should cause you to cancel your workout. Of course, certain times of the year will be busier than others. This is yet another reason for periodization, scheduling your training so that the easiest training weeks correspond with the most stressful weeks of the year.

Reward Yourself for Being Efficient

If you plan to finish a task in a certain period of time and you finish on time, if not early, reward yourself. It does not matter whether the task is related to bodybuilding or not. Treat yourself to a cup of gourmet coffee, go to a different gym for a unique workout, or buy yourself the latest copy of your favorite muscle magazine. It is more than just a break from work. The reward

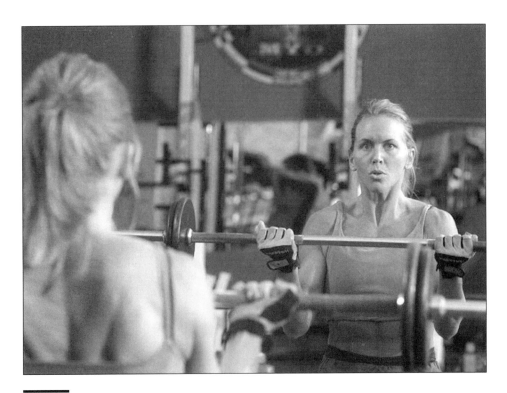

Time management during your workouts will enable you to maintain focus and to maximize your potential.

that you give yourself should be relaxing and reflect your accomplishment of efficient time management.

Reduce Time Sensitivity

Bodybuilders are better attuned to their bodies than most people. Learn to read your body's need for sleep, exercise, food, and intellectual thought. For example, if you are feeling wide awake one night, use that time to wade through difficult paperwork or read a particularly challenging book. If you are feeling sluggish, use that time to relax or go the gym for a workout. Do not be a slave to your watch. Learn to ignore the clock and do what is best for your body.

This may mean adding more flexibility into your workout schedule. For example, you could plan to work out on Monday, Wednesday, and Friday but not at a predetermined time. That way, you will have the structure of knowing which day you will be working out but also the flexibility to work out when it is most convenient.

Use of a Training Partner

Most bodybuilders prefer the commitment, motivation, and enjoyment they get from having a training partner. Training partners will fall into one of two categories: (1) a partner who is interested in your development and looks for ways to help motivate you and guide you toward achieving your goals, or (2) a partner who has no desire to see you reach your bodybuilding goals and whom you must continually motivate. In other words, training partners either enhance or hinder your training. There is no such thing as a neutral training partner. Be sure that yours falls into the first category, not the second.

Of course, the training partnership is a reciprocal exchange of influence: you influence your training partner and your partner influences you. This exchange of influence can have a significant impact on your training effectiveness as well as your enjoyment. When one person has more influence than the other, the situation is less than optimal. Let's face it, all of us have had training partners who enhanced our training and other partners who were almost useless. The ideal situation is to have a training partner that treats their body development with the same level of passion and commitment as you do. You want your training partner to be able to make a valuable contribution to your muscular development in the same way that you want to be able to help them.

Like a coach, your training partner should provide training tips, help you identify your weaknesses, and provide motivation and emotional support during critical moments in your training. Likewise, he or she will be looking to you for the same. The optimal situation is one in which both partners are able to communicate effectively and each person is equally influential.

Knowing Your Partner

Have you ever noticed that when some bodybuilders train together, they seem to have a lot of fun? Have you noticed some bodybuilding partners who seem to know each other's needs so well that they can really motivate each other? Elite bodybuilders who have trained with partners for many years know exactly what their partners need, when to push them through a tough set and when to advise a light set. Admirers of this training harmony may believe that it comes with little effort, that it happens between some people but not others. This could not be farther from the truth. Good training partners, first and foremost, become knowledgeable about the sport of bodybuilding. They also put a lot of energy and time into learning the strengths, weaknesses, and training likes and dislikes of their partners. The good news is, this ability to "train as one" is attainable if you make the effort to learn about bodybuilding and get to know your training partner.

Do you know everything about your partner you should? Do you believe that you understand your partner's feelings, bodybuilding struggles, emotions, psychological outlook, and physical attributes? Do you know your partner's goals? Likewise, do you believe that your partner understands your needs and is comfortable with you? Complete exercise 8.5 to determine how much you know about your partner. (Your partner should also answer these questions.) Then show your responses to your partner and ask him or her for feedback.

Take the time to get to know your partner well, and be open and honest so that your partner can know you. Do your part to ensure that your relationship is one in which every shared opinion is trusted and respected. Being an effective training partner requires taking an active leadership role and encouraging your partner to improve himself or herself. Set an example by improving your own coaching skills. He or she will likely follow.

Communicating Effectively

The importance of effective communication is highlighted in every magazine article, newspaper story, or self-help book on human relationships. Because the way training partners relate to each other is so important, good communication is crucial. Not only will effective communication help improve your workout efficiency and results, it can alleviate, if not prevent, many of the problems that arise between bodybuilders. To get the most out of each training session, it is important that bodybuilding partners build trust and respect. This process begins with opening the lines of communication, being patient, being a good listener, and trying to learn as much as possible about each other.

Communication is a dynamic process. It continually changes in response to a situation and can take many forms. For example, communication can be interpersonal (verbal or nonverbal), intrapersonal (self-talk), written (books, newspapers, magazines, charts, diagrams, and so on), auditory (radio, music), or visual (photographs, modeling, film, video, and so on). Because people express themselves in so many different ways, honest communication is crucial. In other words, what you say should match what you do. For example, if you say that you are happy, you should have a smile on your face, and whatever you write should indicate that you are happy.

To develop good communication with your training partner, you must maintain a good working relationship with each other in and out of the gym. Some of the best training partners are those who form a special bond that extends beyond the gym. This is especially true in times when trust is needed. You must also become supportive of your partner. If your training is to be effective and you are to achieve the goals you have established, you and your partner will have to make sacrifices. Because you will spend so much time together, any strain or discomfort in the relationship will become evident in your workout efficiency.

Every training situation will be an opportunity to improve your communication skills, including expressing your feelings, communicating clearly, being assertive, and listening well. After reading this chapter you now have the knowledge and tools to help you or other bodybuilders you know break through training plateaus. First, you must understand what motivates you

What Do You Know About Your Training Partner?

1. What is your partner's name, age, and gender?

   _____

   _____

2. How many years has your partner been training? Bodybuilding? In competition?

   _____

   _____

   _____

3. How long have you been training with your partner? When did you first start training together?

   _____

   _____

   _____

4. In order of preference, list the five favorite exercises of you and your partner.

   _____

   _____

   _____

   _____

   _____

5. What are your best three body parts? What are your partner's? Which body parts does he or she work out the most?

   _____

   _____

   _____

   _____

   _____

   _____

6. Describe the training sessions you have with your partner. Are they filled with tension or laughter, or are they quiet and professional? Are you happy with your training and muscular development? What about your partner?

_____

_____

_____

7. How would you describe your partner's body (bulky, ripped, symmetrical, smooth, tight, loose, and so on)? How would your partner describe your body?

_____

_____

_____

8. What do you think your strengths and weaknesses are? Would your partner agree with you? What are your partner's strengths and weaknesses?

_____

_____

_____

_____

9. What are your nutritional habits? What are your partner's? What are his or her three food temptations? What advice would you give your partner about nutrition? What advice would you give yourself?

_____

_____

_____

_____

10. What lifestyle changes could you and your training partner make to enhance muscular development?

_____

_____

_____

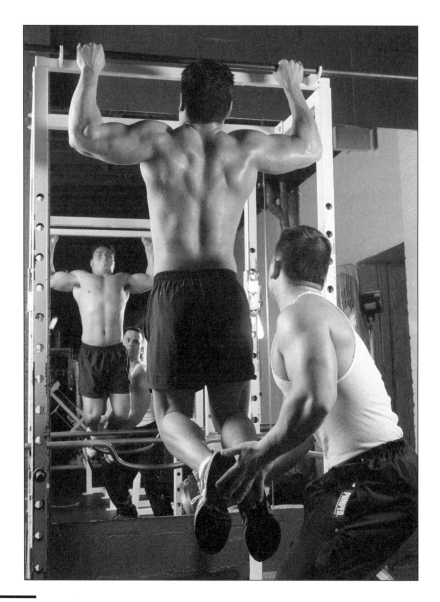

Communicating with your partner helps both of you to get the most out of each training session.

to engage in bodybuilding and what it will take for you to continue. Once you have an understanding of your own motivation, you can apply some of the strategies in this chapter designed to help you break through training plateaus. Finally, getting a training partner is an important step to overcoming the inertia in a training program. Breaking through training plateaus is possible for you and every other bodybuilder. It just takes a concerted effort to think with your head and dream with your heart.

CHAPTER 9

Mindful Bodybuilding for Women

Heidi Paa

Imagine a crowded weight room. Everywhere you look, people are bench pressing, doing squats, curling dumbbells, and dead-lifting. The room is surrounded by mirrors and filled with plates, ropes, pulleys, and other "toys" used to pummel muscle into submission. A combination of sweat and chalk, remnants of the last set and perhaps a personal best, weighs down the air. Thrashing music plays on the radio, interrupted by spotters encouraging their partners to push through lifts. Veins are popping, sweat is dripping, and weights are clanging as bodybuilders push through one more rep, 10 more pounds, to finish that last set.

Look around the room. How many women do you see? Years ago, the answer would be none. In fact, years ago many weight-training gyms did not even have women's locker rooms. Why would they? It was absurd to think that a woman would want to engage in such a "manly" activity. Women worked out in so-called fitness centers, vibrating fat off their hips and performing donkey kicks by the thousands.

Fortunately, this picture has changed. Although men still dominate most weight rooms and far too many women limit their physical activity to countless hours of cardiovascular work, women are increasingly incorporating strength training into their fitness programs. Women are also becoming serious weight trainers, evidenced by the number of female bodybuilders, fitness competitors, and powerlifters. Female athletes of all levels are realizing the performance-enhancing effects of strength training. Strong women such as Serena Williams, Dara Torres, and Gabrielle Reece proudly show off the fruits of their labor and empower other women to "hit the metal."

Finding their membership becoming increasingly female, gym owners are trying to make their establishments women friendly. For example, many gyms across the country have developed "women only" weight rooms to welcome the growing number of women who are interested in strength training but may feel intimidated by the overwhelming male presence in most weight rooms. These "women only" weight rooms have sparked heated debates about sexual discrimination and gender stereotyping. Despite the controversy surrounding them, however, "women only" areas evidence a female migration into weight rooms that is not showing any signs of slowing down.

This chapter is intended to address issues unique to female bodybuilders and should be considered a supplement to the rest of the book.

Why Do Women Weight Train?

What is behind this female migration? What is attracting women to the dumbbells and barbells? In general, society's awareness of weight training and its health benefits has increased. The media has begun to publicize the role that strength training plays in reducing blood pressure, total cholesterol, and body fat composition, as well as its role in slowing the natural decline in strength and mobility that comes with age. The addition of strength training to the American College of Sports and Medicine (ACSM) guidelines for physical activity has also increased the popularity of weight training, for both women and men. Women, in particular, are discovering that weight training offers a number of unique physiological and psychological benefits unparalleled by other activities.

Physiological Benefits

Women's lives are becoming increasingly demanding. Women with full-time careers and young children find themselves juggling numerous responsibilities both in and outside the home. As women increase muscle strength, their bodies become more prepared to perform daily activities such as lifting children and groceries, or enduring long days at work. This increase in muscle strength can also protect women from various physical conditions. Weight training produces

- increased bone density, a protective factor against osteoporosis, which affects up to 40 percent of post-menopausal women;
- stronger ligaments, which may help prevent muscle imbalances and preventing knee problems, a condition women are more prone to;
- increased upper body strength, as women usually have weaker upper bodies compared to their lower bodies; and
- increased endurance, which helps to prevent inactivity and a sedentary lifestyle, an increasing problem in today's society.

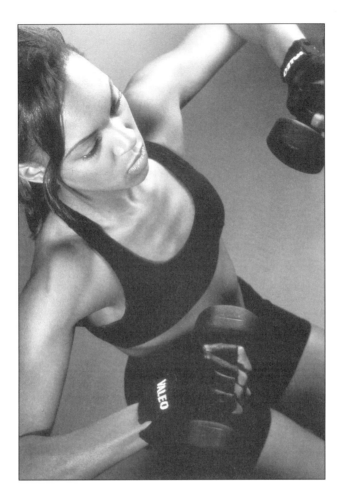

For women, weight training doesn't just lead to physical changes; stronger muscles yield stronger minds.

Psychological Benefits

While the physiological benefits are important, perhaps the greatest benefits are psychological. Along with the supple, muscular physique produced by serious bodybuilding comes an inner strength. Though not a cure-all for every problem, the improvement in psychological health that accompanies weight training can have profound effects in the lives of female bodybuilders. Among them are the following:

• Increased confidence. Most women find that weight training offers a sense of accomplishment that transcends the gym. As women's muscles become strong, they also feel stronger internally, better equipped to handle life's challenges. The difference between trying and not trying, succeeding and not succeeding, is usually not ability but confidence. Being able to say

"I can" to a set of heavy squats translates to being able to say "I can and I will" to other challenges at home, work, or school.

• Increased self-esteem. As women grow strong physically, they begin to like themselves more. In our culture, low self-esteem is at epidemic proportions among women. Indeed, more women have been diagnosed with depression than ever before. Whether these statistics are representative of a real problem or a society that is more likely to label women as depressed, the fact that women are increasingly failing to find value in themselves cannot be denied. Bodybuilding is one way women can discover their psychological strength and learn to embrace it. Through lifting weights, women begin to view themselves differently, and they begin to like what they see.

• Improved body image. Most women are socialized from girlhood to hate their bodies. This is no doubt influenced by the unrealistic body ideals presented by the media and the objectification of women in our culture. At an alarmingly young age, girls learn that their worth is measured by their physical appearance and that the only acceptable body shape is the overly slim, often emaciated, physique idolized by the media. Unfortunately, for more than 90 percent of women, this physique is unobtainable, which puts women in the lifelong cycle of body hatred that can lead to eating disorders.

Although not immune to body dissatisfaction and eating disorders, female bodybuilders often come to appreciate and even like their bodies. Some strong women actually become comfortable discussing their unique physical strengths, such as well-developed quads or wide backs. Indeed, the basic philosophy behind strength training could serve to protect women from falling victim to the self-destructive cycle of body hatred.[1] Weight lifting requires a body that is well-nourished and able to undergo the rigors of training. In addition, bodybuilders value physiques that have well-developed, mature muscles groomed through years of hard work.

• Decreased risk of disordered eating. This argument recently found scientific support.[2] Researchers combined a number of studies on the relationship between athletic participation and eating disorders in women to look for trends. In general, results suggested that female athletes were less likely to experience eating disorders than nonathletic women. This was particularly evident among high school athletes. Although dancers and participants in elite sports that emphasize a lean physique (for example, gymnastics) reported a higher incidence of eating disorders, participation in nonelite sports served as a buffer for young women. That is, young women who participated in nonelite sports were actually less likely to develop eating disorders compared to their peers who did not play sports. According to researchers, participation in athletics for fitness, fun, and even social interaction might be quite valuable, especially for girls. Given that women often participate in bodybuilding for these very reasons, it seems possible that bodybuilding might help to prevent negative body image and eating disorders.

• Decreased stress and fatigue. Research has proven the role that physical activity plays in helping to manage stress and increase energy levels. In contrast to ineffective coping strategies such as substance abuse and overeating, weight training is a healthy, effective way for women to cope with their increasingly stressful lives. It is called "resistance training," after all. Moreover, engaging in an intense, physically taxing activity like bodybuilding may serve a cathartic purpose for women who otherwise would not express feelings of anger and resentment.

A body that is strong and healthy is better equipped to handle stressful life events. The muscles developed through weight training can literally become energizing forces providing an overall sense of vitality and strength.

• Empowerment. The media often depicts women as passive, weak creatures with thin, frail bodies. In American culture, for that matter, passivity among women has been reinforced. Indeed, women in powerful positions are called "bitches," while women in subservient roles are called "sweet" and "caring." While it is true that women often excel at nurturing, they may do so at their own peril. In addition to increasing their physical power, bodybuilding may also help women to become mentally powerful. Female bodybuilders simultaneously recognize their physical strengths and limitations. Through this process, women become aware of the limits in their own lives, thus empowering themselves to say no when necessary.

• Creative self-expression. Many women begin bodybuilding for physical reasons, for example, to increase muscle mass and strength. As their muscles change, however, so does their motivation for training. What likely began as a way to change their external selves, their bodies, becomes a conduit for expressing parts of their internal selves, such as their creativity. Through trying different exercises and training methods, women learn to "sculpt" their muscles and to view their strong bodies as a symbol for who they are on the inside. Through this self-expression, women may find it easier to connect to their creative energies in other aspects of their lives.

• Increased self-care. As noted earlier, women engage in a number of activities and fulfill a number of different roles, including girlfriend or life partner, mother or grandmother, employer or employee, home manager, friend, sister, chef, and so on. Because women so often find themselves caring for everyone in their lives but themselves, feelings of resentment, disconnection, and dissatisfaction can arise. Fortunately, women are learning the importance of self-care. (Incidentally, this term did not even exist 10 years ago.) Today, thankfully, self-help books and popular media encourage women to schedule time to care for themselves, just as they schedule other daily tasks.

The philosophy behind the self-care movement is that women cannot effectively fulfill their other roles unless they feel physically, psychologically, and spiritually equipped to do so. Therefore, women must put their own self-care ahead of everything else. Although simplistic, this is a far cry from the

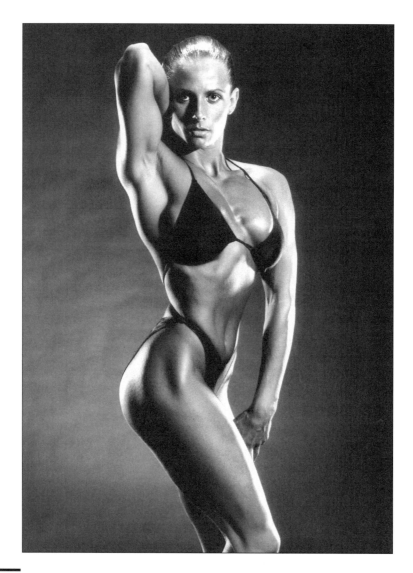

Women receive many messages that tell them to be ashamed of their bodies, but weight-training can help them to accept and embrace the shape of their bodies.

priority many women assign their own needs, even the most basic needs such as adequate sleep.

Scheduling a trip to the gym or making an appointment with a personal trainer can be an excellent reminder of the importance of self-care. Many women refer to their weight-training sessions as "me time," that is, time when they can ignore other demands and focus solely on themselves. Because of the self-oriented, mental concentration involved in bodybuilding, increased attention and awareness of self-care is a natural result. Women need only look in one of the countless mirrors at the gym for a reminder of why they are there.

How Should Women Weight Train?

If you are reading this book, you probably already enjoy lifting weights. Whether it be for bodybuilding, powerlifting, or general health, you are no stranger to the iron. Therefore, this section does not detail such elementary principles of starting a weight-training program as proper technique and sample exercises. Instead, this section outlines more advanced, psychologically oriented information related to weight training for women.

Setting Realistic Training Goals

As noted in previous chapters, both male and female bodybuilders should use long- and short-term goals that are specific, measurable, and challenging but obtainable. Unfortunately, many women find this process difficult. For example, because the ultraskinny female physique so pervasive in the media is touted as the ideal body image, women often start bodybuilding with a long-term goal that is unrealistic for their body type. Many women do not allow enough time to achieve their goal. This leaves many female bodybuilders feeling discouraged, thinking they have failed, and they stop training.

Women looking to emulate the looks of the professional female bodybuilders and fitness competitors in muscle magazines can also get discouraged easily. Seeing these ripped physiques, many women incorrectly assume that these models look that way all the time. In reality, competitors schedule photo shoots near contest times, and models usually diet for weeks before their own photo shoots. Although muscular physiques are at least more accurate than the very thin, tall physiques with little muscle and even less fat presented in mainstream media, to women bodybuilders, these images can still be a constant reminder that they are physical failures, that their own bodies are not beautiful.

Even professional female bodybuilders have difficulty watching their bodies change from very lean to a normal level of body fat after a contest. After the cutting period, when they drastically reduce their body fat, what once felt like a normal level of body fat may feel very fat. Indeed, for many professional female bodybuilders, unrealistic expectations can be just as big a struggle as they are for most women.

Without a doubt, the most damaging consequence of setting unrealistic goals and measuring your appearance by media images is the vicious and pervasive cycle of body hatred. If you asked women to name something they like about their bodies, most would be hard pressed to come up with something. If you asked them to discuss their physical "flaws," however, they would probably talk your ear off! Especially young women are heard to say, "I hate my thighs," or "I look so fat in these pants."

At best, body hatred turns to feeling inadequate as a person; at worst, it turns to self-hatred. The result: overwhelming numbers of women struggle with diet, negative body image, poor self-esteem, and obsession with food, exercise, and weight loss. Before female bodybuilders set training goals, it is essential that they examine their attitudes about their bodies. Having unrealistic expectations or negative body esteem will lead to unrealistic or inappropriate goals.

Listening to your own self-talk will reveal most of your personal attitudes about your body shape. What do you tell yourself about your body? Are you realistic, encouraging, negative, or berating? Do you associate your worth as a person with how you feel about your body? Answer the questions in exercise 9.1 to identify your body-related self-talk. If you discover that your relationship with your body could use some improvement, start with the following three steps. If you want to explore this issue in greater depth, individual and group counseling, community workshops, and self-help books might be useful.

1. First and foremost, you must accept the physique you inherited from your parents. Bodies vary genetically in size, composition, and ability to gain muscle. This is not a bad thing! Difference is the basis of uniqueness and individuality. It adds complexity to our world. Just as differences in attitudes allow debate, innovation, and creativity, differences in body shape enable athletic competition, distribution of work, and physical attraction.

Although physiques can be transformed through weight training and dieting, each person is born with a certain body type. This genetic "blue-print," which determines body shape and size, will never change. Take the calf muscles as an example. Genetically, some bodybuilders have long, full calves that easily take on that "diamond" appearance. Other bodybuilders' calves are short, making it more difficult for these muscles to appear full. Yes, with hard and consistent training, calf muscles can become larger. But some bodybuilders will never possess the full, triangular calves that so many bodybuilders seek. In the words of author Sarah Ban Breathnach, "If you can't be with the body you love, love the body you're with."[3]

2. You must understand and accept that the physical ideal presented in the media is not only unrealistic for the majority of women; it is unhealthy. Too many women waste hours of physical and psychological energy attempting to reach this unattainable goal. It is impossible to maintain presentation shape all year and add muscle at the same time.

If looking at unrealistically lean women causes you to feel bad about your body, stop looking! Instead, read a book or listen to motivational tapes. Moreover, rather than aspire to look like a magazine model, who was most likely enhanced and airbrushed by computer, aspire to look like the best version of yourself, not someone else. Personal trainers, training partners, and friends can serve as objective support during your bodybuilding process. Ask them to look at your goals and offer feedback as to whether they are realistic.

3. You must recognize and celebrate the parts of your body that you like. The socialization of women does not generally include learning to

Exercise 9.1   How Do You Feel About Your Body?

To help you explore your thoughts and feelings about your body, answer the following questions honestly. Try to answer them quickly and avoid thinking excessively. Trust your first instinct.

1. What do I tell myself about my body when I wake up in the morning?

2. When among other women what do I tell myself about my body or my weight?

3. How do I react when people compliment me on one of my physical features?

4. When was the last time I allowed myself to think something positive about my body?

5. What image best represents how I talk to myself about my body (e.g., an evil witch, a best friend, a coach)?

---

recognize personal strengths. When coupled with the pervasive body hatred among women, no wonder it is so difficult for women to find anything they like about their bodies!

During your workouts, use the compliments you get from others as "stepping stones" to compliment yourself. Every body has at least one strength. Find yours and acknowledge it. Likewise, recognize and celebrate your body's uniqueness. Answer the questions in exercise 9.2 to begin the process of recognizing and appreciating your physical strengths.

Exercise 9.2   Learning to Like Your Body

Answer the questions below as a way to begin thinking and talking about your body in a supportive, positive way. You may have more than one response per question. That's great—the more, the better.

1. What is my favorite body part to train? Why?

2. What is my strongest body part?

3. What do I like most about my body? Why?

4. What body part am I most proud of? Why?

5. Tell yourself something positive about each of your body parts—face, neck, shoulders, pecs, breasts, arms, abdomen, glutes, thighs, calves, feet, and so on. Include any features that you would like to specify.

Achieving Bodybuilding Goals

Popular fitness magazines and even scientific journals contain conflicting information about women and weight training. For example, although some fitness experts advocate different training programs for women and men, others believe that muscle is muscle, claiming there is no reason that women and men should train differently. In addition, for fear of getting "too big," many women use lighter weights and more reps to build strength. With so many differing opinions—many might call them "myths"—many women are confused about the correct way to reach their bodybuilding goals. This section explores these training myths and offers suggestions for deciding on

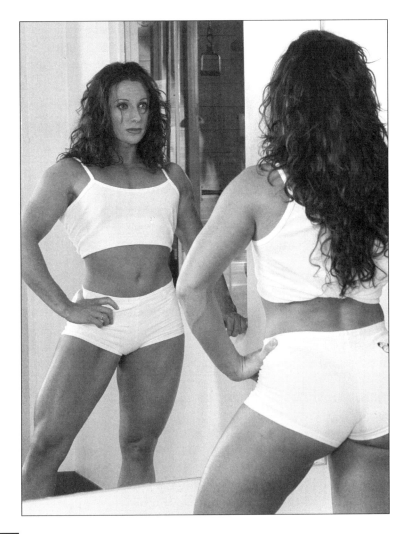

Does looking in the mirror trigger negative thoughts about your body? Use bodybuilding to construct a more positive body image.

your own. After you've completed this exercise, use the goal-setting information in chapter 8 to further outline your bodybuilding goals.

Myth 1: Women who train with heavy weights will quickly develop large muscles.

"I don't want to get too big," beginning female weight trainers often say to their trainers. After seeing images of female bodybuilders in popular fitness magazines (many who are hormonally-enhanced), many women incorrectly assume that a very muscular physique is within their genetic potential. In reality, women need to train quite intensely and for several years to develop muscularity. Because women lack the higher levels of testosterone found in men, their muscles develop more slowly and they simply cannot achieve a comparable amount of muscle size. A majority of successful female body-builders are near or past the age of 30 and have been training with heavy weights for a long, long time. To be sure, an increase in muscular size is no accident in female bodybuilders. As many female bodybuilders will tell you, usually with a laugh, "I wish adding muscle were that easy."

Myth 2: Women and men with similar training goals should train differently.

If you take a quick look through the fitness section of a popular bookstore, you will see a number of weight-training books geared specifically toward women. While the existence of these books points to the need for different training for men and women, a comparison of actual exercises will reveal few, if any, differences. Both types of books advocate the same basic exercises used by most bodybuilders: bench presses, military presses, squats, lunges, and so on.

Of course, this does not mean that women's weight-training books are of no value. Indeed, they often contain photos of women demonstrating each exercise and information on issues specifically related to women, such as eating disorders. In addition, seeing photos of women weight training and reading bodybuilding books written by women may provide encourage-ment and motivation. But the exercises advocated to building muscle are usually quite similar to other, more gender-neutral books.

Dr. Mariah Liggett holds a PhD in exercise physiology as well as 13 world and national powerlifting titles and four world powerlifting records. Accord-ing to Dr. Liggett, if women's and men's goals are similar, women should train no differently than men. For example, a woman wanting to gain size should train no differently than a man wanting to gain size: both should emphasize basic, compound exercises that target major muscle groups, using progres-sively heavier weights for no more than 10 reps. Liggett, who has been powerlifting for more than 20 years, was the first woman to dead-lift over 300 pounds and has helped both male and female powerlifters prepare for competition, "Based on both personal experience and scientific literature, I would coach a woman no differently than I would coach a man." In fact, all of Dr. Liggett's pre-competition training partners have been men. "I prefer to train with someone stronger," she says. "It motivates me to catch up."

Myth 3: Toning and sculpting muscle are different from building muscle.

When applied to muscle, the words *tone* and *sculpt* are synonymous with the word *build*. In other words, there is no difference between toning a muscle and building a muscle: both are achieved through the process of progressive overload. Realizing that many women are afraid to "build" their bodies (see myth 1), the fitness industry began to use terms like *body sculpt* and *muscle tone* to trick women into thinking they were not building muscle. There is

Strong, Healthy, and Feminine: Gina Masoni

Although a newcomer to the world of bodybuilding, Gina Masoni is already getting attention for her symmetrical physique and dedicated work ethic. After attending numerous bodybuilding shows, Gina was attracted to the muscular physique and yearned for her chance to be on stage. Since that time, she has competed in four shows and plans to continue her bodybuilding career in natural competitions. Known for her incredible strength and determination in the gym, Gina offers the following words of wisdom to other women.

1. "Stay natural!" Amid pressure to take steroids to enhance her physique, Gina has vowed to remain a natural competitor. "I've seen what steroids do to women," she says, "and I feel strongly that it's not worth it." In her short bodybuilding career, Gina has made significant gains in muscle size without drugs, and she plans to continue on this path: "I became a bodybuilder to stay healthy, happy, and strong. I'd like to be a positive role model for women."

2. "Enjoy the process." Gina loves doing heavy squats just as much as she loves standing on stage. She says, "success in bodybuilding does not come overnight. It takes time to build muscle—you need to be patient and take your time." Bodybuilders who do not enjoy the process of building muscle will not last long in the sport. Before a contest, Gina visualizes how she wants her physique to look and uses that image for motivation. She enjoys watching her strength increase and allows herself to feel good about even the smallest progress.

3. "Train hard!" Gina has learned though many hours of training that well-developed muscles do not come easily. "Despite what many women think, you need to train very intensely to add muscle," she says. Gina has also learned the benefits of regularly setting goals. In addition to setting long-term, competition-related goals, Gina sets goals for every workout: "I always push myself to go heavier while also paying attention to my form. I rely on training partners for motivation and feedback on my technique."

simply no difference between a muscle that is toned and a muscle that is built, and they are both achieved with similar methods.

Myth 4: Bodybuilding is a man's sport.

Although most experienced female bodybuilders feel very comfortable among the heavy iron, look at the face of a beginner as she walks toward the free weights. She is probably afraid of looking stupid, of others talking about her, of not knowing what she is doing, and so on. Not only that, but just being in the presence of so many strong people, male and female, can be over-whelming to a beginner. It is no coincidence that women limit strength training to using weight machines, which allow them to work their muscles and, at the same time, avoid the free weight area.

With time, however, most women come to find their fears of the weight room irrational. In reality, once you get to know them, bodybuilders are usually down-to-earth people. Besides, they are probably more interested in the amount of protein they got during their last meal than who the new person in the gym is. More often than not, the weight room becomes a place where women feel not only comfortable but strong, confident, and empow-ered as well.

A Word About Nutrition

Although food and nutrition are addressed in chapter 4, this chapter would not be complete without addressing the complex relationship many women

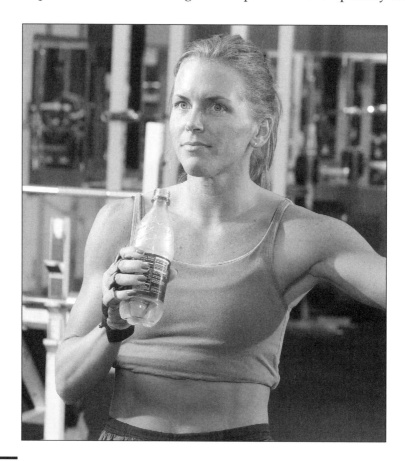

Female bodybuilders understand the importance of good nutrition in developing their muscular physiques.

have with food. Many women connect emotionally with food. Using it as a coping mechanism, they turn to food for comfort when they are anxious, lonely, sad, and even happy. Even though the bodybuilding lifestyle emphasizes muscle-building nutrition, female bodybuilders are not immune from having unhealthy relationships with food. For example, competitive bodybuilders, male and female, frequently celebrate the end of their contest diets by eating a large quantity of high-calorie foods, sometimes for days.

Because society puts such importance on women's appearance, when women do not measure up to the physical ideal, they often believe that they do not possess value in their current physical condition. Like any person, male or female, who feels undervalued or unvalued, women use whatever means possible to change the way they are perceived by others. All too often, these means include drastic and dangerous dieting. Indeed, the "normalization of dieting" has reached epidemic proportions among women and young girls in this country. Up to 50 percent of fourth-grade girls report that they are currently on a diet and research shows that the majority of women (and girls), regardless of their weight, think they are fat and are currently trying to lose weight.

The bodybuilding culture may protect women from falling into this diet trap. The phrase that has taken root in the mainstream—"You can never be too thin"—has no place in the bodybuilding world. Women wanting to make gains in muscle size quickly learn that a malnourished body progresses slowly, if at all. The popular phrase, "You have to eat big to get big" applies to women as well as men! In stark contrast to the popular media images of frail women, female bodybuilders often feel proud of their large muscles.

Jean Kilbourne is well known for her all-out attack on the advertising industry. She was the first to illustrate the negative impact of advertising on women with her award-winning documentary, *Killing Us Softly,* a shocking film that examined the portrayal of women in media. In her most recent book, *Deadly Persuasion: Why Women and Girls Must Fight the Addictive Power of Advertising,*[4] Kilbourne argues that advertising encourages people to form relationships with objects (cookies, cars, shampoo, and so on) by subtly convincing them that they need these things to be happy. Think about the last five advertisements you saw on television or in a magazine. Most, if not all, of them probably conveyed the message that by using the product advertised, you could become more attractive, release tension, improve relationships, be more successful, be more desirable—the possibilities are endless.

Like other objects in advertising, according to Kilbourne, many food advertisements contain images of women using food for an emotional purpose. Rather than a substance that keeps bodies healthy and strong, food is portrayed as a prize, a comfort, an ever-present best friend. Think about dessert advertisements. Most involve women rewarding themselves with chocolate, candy, or some other sugar-laden food. Rather than rewarding themselves with internal validation, feelings of accomplishment and pride,

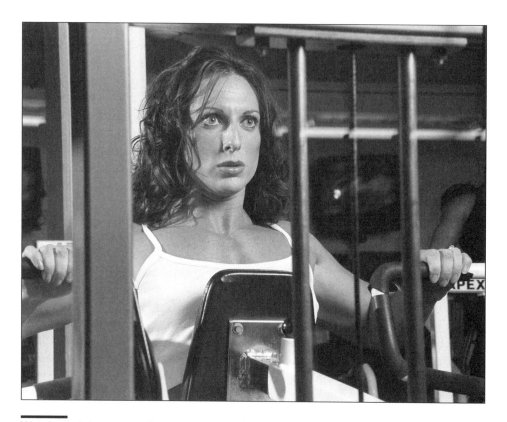

Weight-training can relieve stress and help stop cycles of overeating when over-whelmed.

women are shown turning to an external source (food) for validation. These ads, specifically targeted toward women, encourage women to connect with food rather than their bodies and minds. If you think this type of advertising is aimed at men too, try to recall the last time you saw a commercial that featured a man eating chocolate ice cream while saying, "I deserve this."

Advertising also encourages women to cope with uncomfortable emotions such as sadness, anger, and isolation by eating. Dessert ads suggest that eating a rich chocolate cake can take away the pressure and stress of negative or painful life experiences. Ads such as these reinforce the socialization of women, which discourages their feeling and expressing negative emotions. With repeated exposure to such images and societal attitudes, many women learn to "numb" themselves with food rather than connect and cope with "unacceptable" emotions.

Because emotionally connecting with food is so common among women, female bodybuilders may have difficulty determining if their relationships with food are problematic. In general, if you find yourself repeatedly using food for emotional purposes or if your relationship with food negatively affects your relationship with yourself or loved ones, you may want to examine the role that food plays in your life. Individual and group therapy provide an excellent forum for exploring your relationship with food and beginning to build a healthier connection with yourself and others.

Putting It All Together

One purpose of this chapter is to emphasize the profound internal and external rewards women can reap from bodybuilding. In addition to increases in muscularity and physical strength, through bodybuilding, women can also build themselves internally, resulting in increases in psychological strength. Hopefully, this chapter has helped you put words to the feelings you have when you train and as you become stronger. Most likely, you have been reading this chapter and saying to yourself, "Yes, bodybuilding makes me feel that way" and "Yes, I agree with that." You are living testimony to the relationship between building muscle and building confidence and self-esteem.

In closing, I offer a challenge to the many strong women who will read this book. Now that you have experienced the powerful impact of bodybuilding, your next challenge is to pass your knowledge on to other women and welcome them into the weight room. Not only can you dispel the numerous myths about women and weight training, you can also show women how bodybuilding can foster an empowering journey within. You can serve as a mentor to women who are new to weight training and provide support as they try something new and become stronger.

Dr. Mariah Liggett and Carol Semple-Marzetta both feel an obligation to pass their knowledge and expertise on to women. "In every area of life, including the gym," Liggett says, "people need a supportive social network." A world-class powerlifter and fitness center director of Compuserve headquarters, Dr. Liggett encourages others to strive toward their own fitness goals. Ms. Semple-Marzetta agrees: "When I became interested in bodybuilding, I approached two women in my gym who trained very hard and asked if I could work out with them. With their help, I learned how to train correctly and build the muscle necessary to excel in fitness competitions. I would like to serve in a similar role for other women."

Now it is your turn. Smile and say "hello" to that new woman as she enters the weight room. Compliment a fellow bodybuilder on her strength or muscle size. Invite a woman to train with you for a few weeks. The next time any woman asks you about your diet "secrets," tell her how good weightlifting makes you feel on the inside, in addition to the results on the outside. There are countless ways you can share your passion for bodybuilding. Some female bodybuilders become personal trainers and get a paycheck for sharing their knowledge and skills. You need not expend a great deal of time and energy to make a difference. What is important is that you do what feels most natural to you, and that you do something.

CHAPTER 10

Sharpening the Mind While Sculpting the Body

Have you ever thought of yourself as an artist, a creator of image? Artists need a sharp mind to pay special attention to detail as they paint, draw, or mold their art form. Just like an artist, you will need to engage your brain as you religiously work on the canvas of your body. The better you can sharpen your mind and focus on the task at hand, the more quickly you will develop the body you desire. Understanding the role that arousal regulation, focus, distraction control, and visualization skills play in successful bodybuilding will provide you with the mental clarity essential to bodybuilding success.

Body Awareness

Body awareness is concerned with the mind-body relationship and understanding this dynamic connection is a critical component of bodybuilding success. It is the first step toward relaxation, distraction control, and visualization. The better connected your mind and body the more responsive you will be to physical training. Unfortunately, more often than not, one component in the mind-body relationship is emphasized to the detriment of the other. Have you ever said, "The best thing I can do is ignore my thoughts," or "If I put my mind to it, I can make my body do anything?" These are both unhealthy statements.

An essential component of a solid mind-body connection is the way that you feel mentally and physically. Your mental and physical feelings provide you with a keen sense of awareness that enables you to identify with the mental, physical, and emotional sides of you. Though a lot of this is learned from experience, you can enhance this learning process through various techniques of body awareness training.

Remember that an amazingly sophisticated relationship exists between your nervous system and your body. As you train, thousands of signals are being sent to your brain. Your brain then makes decisions and sends signals back through the nervous system to be broken down into simpler and more precise messages for each muscle fiber. The point is that a complicated relationship exists between your brain and your working muscles. Therefore, it is clear that the more developed your body awareness the more you will get out of a workout. Learn to listen to what your body is telling your brain and what your brain is telling your body. As you do, you will be better able to mentally prepare (i.e., relax, visualize, or energize) for intense training sessions and for bodybuilding shows and competitions.

Body Awareness Exercises

The following exercises have been adapted from *Sporting Body Sporting Mind.*[1]

EXERCISE 10.1 NONVISUAL PRACTICE

Think of an exercise that you can perform with your eyes closed (for example, biceps curls).

1. Perform the skill with your eyes open as you would normally perform it.
2. Now perform the same skill several times with your eyes closed. Having been taught to use mirrors in training, this is strange for most bodybuilders. Nevertheless, you must learn to rely on your non-visual senses.
3. Become aware of how each movement feels, what you hear, and how you use your nonvisual senses in performing each movement.
4. Shift between having your eyes open and closed several times until you begin to get a kinaesthetic awareness of the skill.
5. Finish the exercise, keeping your eyes open for the final set. (Note: This body awareness exercise is also useful for breaking through training plateaus.)

EXERCISE 10.2 COLORED BODY PARTS

This simple exercise increases body awareness and adds another dimension to mental rehearsal.

1. Close your eyes and relax. In your imagination, set the scene for a particular exercise you want to perform and watch yourself performing the set.

2. Imagine that you see each area of your body surrounded by a color: primary muscle groups are red, secondary muscle groups are blue, and muscle groups not involved in the exercise are green. If you were to imagine yourself doing a set of incline bench presses, you would see the pectoralis major, anterior deltoid, and the triceps colored in red, the pectoralis minor and the medial and posterior heads of the deltoid in blue, and the rest of the muscle groups in green.

This technique is a great way to isolate the different parts of your body as you mentally rehearse the set, and it allows you to attune more closely to those body parts. It may also help you to pinpoint more specifically the influence that certain muscle groups have on the performance of the set.

EXERCISE 10.3 BODY SCAN

By conducting a body scan, you begin to develop a kinaesthetic awareness of your body. A body scan includes noting sensations of cold and hot, rough and smooth, wet and dry, as well as any internal sensations and signals produced during movement patterns, such as balance, coordination, and the relationship certain body parts have with one another. While bodybuilders are often attuned to these sensations, the body scan can further hone and improve that awareness.

The purpose of this technique is to slowly become attuned to each part of your body, noticing any muscle tension, soreness, numbness, or relaxation. Like many of the exercises presented in this book, the body scan can be practiced almost anywhere and at any time.

If you are sitting, begin the body scan from the head and move downward. If you are lying down, start with your feet and move upward. Concentrate on a specific part of your body, trying to determine all the sensations experienced. Concentrate on each body part for approximately 10 seconds until you have scanned every part of your body.

The following protocol, adapted from *Sporting Body Sporting Mind*, is an excellent example of a body scan progression.[2]

1. Close your eyes and relax. Become aware of your feet and explore how they feel. Can you differentiate your big toe from your fifth toe? Do this with the other foot. What is the difference between your right foot and your left foot? Does one feel larger than the other? Which one do you normally put your weight on while resting?

2. Move your focus to your calves and knees. Which are the main muscles in your calves? How are they attached to your knees? What is the relationship between your knee and ankles? How do your knees

function? Can you feel the kneecap? Can you feel it attached to your knee joint?

3. Focus on your thighs. How tight is the largest muscle on the front of your thighs? What do the backs of your thighs feel like? Can you feel the way in which your thigh muscles relate to those of your buttocks? Do you sense the way that your knees connect to your thighs?

4. Concentrate on your pelvis area. Feel how the various muscles interconnect in order to form your pelvis. Feel the muscles of your buttocks and the muscles of your groin. Can you feel how your pelvis connects to your thighs? How do your hips feel? Can you feel the weight of your body being supported by your buttocks? Are you aware of how your pelvis connects to your abdomen? How about to your lower back?

5. Shift your attention to your abdomen. Feel the muscles of your abdomen. Which ones do you use in your workouts? Imagine for a few moments where your internal organs are: the intestines, the stomach, the liver, and the gall bladder. How do they feel?

6. Slowly move your attention up to your chest and rib cage. Let yourself breathe and as you do observe how your chest and ribs move. Do you feel pressure as you inhale or exhale?

7. Focus on the whole of your back, an area you almost never see. Spend some time concentrating on your upper and lower back, kinaesthetically exploring each area. Mentally review how much of it you can see or cannot see.

8. Turn your attention to your shoulders. Does it feel like your right shoulder is even with the left? Are you aware of how they rest on top of your rib cage? Do you notice your shoulder blades pushing against the ground?

9. Now move your attention down your arms, feeling each section in turn. Notice how your upper arms are connected to your shoulders. Are you aware of how they connect to your elbows? What do your elbows feel like? Consider how they function. Think about your forearms. Can you feel the way that your elbows and wrists are connected?

10. Spend some time feeling your hands and fingers. Wiggle them finger by finger, and then joint by joint. Do all your fingers feel the same? Are any of your fingers sore, tired, or injured?

11. Focus on your neck. Spend time thinking about the front of your neck and the muscles that lead down into your chest and to the top of your sternum. Is the back of your neck tight, relaxed, or sore? Are you aware of how your neck is connected to your shoulders and head? Move your head lightly and notice how your neck feels.

12. Move your attention to your head. Notice each of the areas of your face: your forehead, eyes, cheeks, nose, jaw muscles, chin, lips, tongue,

and the inside of your mouth. Are any of them tight, relaxed, or in pain?

13. When you have completed this inventory, take a couple of minutes to go through your body again, this time spending extra time concentrating on whichever parts of your body feel the least familiar. For example, if the muscles in your legs feel tight, then go back and spend some extra time trying to relax them.

14. Once you have finished the entire body scan, open your eyes and return your attention to the room.

Once you become skilled in conducting a full body scan while sitting or lying down, you can practice it at the gym or on stage. Go through an inventory of your body while you are performing a set such as the seated row. Notice the tension in your wrist and forearms as you hold the grips, the piercing of your eyes as you focus intently on the weight stack, the intensity of your breathing, and the burning sensation in your latissmus dorsi (lats) as you rip off a maximum number of reps. As you become more attuned to your body in the gym, you will begin to see substantial improvement in your lifting technique and muscular development.

Arousal Regulation

There are numerous examples of athletes who have failed or performed poorly in sport simply because they were unable to maintain control throughout the event. As discussed throughout this book, the mind-body connection is highly complex and integrated. Whatever goes on in the mind affects the body, and vice versa.

Obviously, bodybuilders need a certain amount of arousal to accomplish a task. Some need to be mentally "pumped up" to perform at their best, while others need to be calm and relaxed. Believe it or not, more athletes perform poorly as a result of being overaroused than they do as a result of being underaroused. Bodybuilders face a dilemma in this area. In training situations, it is to their advantage to function at a high level of arousal in order to be focused on the workout. In competitions, however, bodybuilders must have control over their thoughts.

Levels of arousal exist on a continuum (see figure 10.1) and are measurable. You can quickly determine your current level of arousal by checking your heart rate, breathing rate, the amount you're sweating, and whether you are experiencing "butterflies" or not. You are likely at your most relaxed state when you are sleeping, but this level of arousal is clearly not appropriate for optimal training performance. Likewise, you may be stressed out just before an important examination, during a difficult situation at work, or minutes before going on stage at a competition, but this level of arousal is also inappropriate for optimal training performance. Whether you are training in the gym or about to go on stage, there is an optimal level of arousal

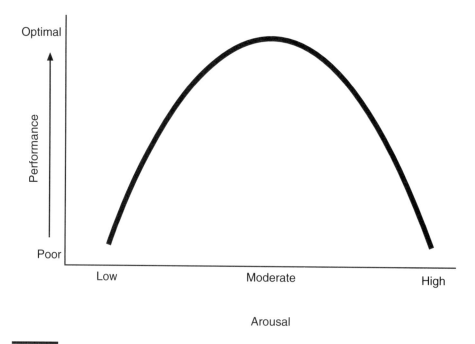

Figure 10.1 The inverted relationship between arousal and performance.

necessary for optimal performance. As a bodybuilder, your challenge is to understand what your optimal level is. Table 10.1 lists emotions and feelings that are typically associated with optimal arousal, overarousal, and underarousal. Check to see if any of the emotions and feelings are similar to your experience during training or competition. The goal should be to experience emotions that are indicative of optimal arousal.

The key to arousal regulation is the ability to relax under pressure and to energize your mind and body when necessary. Regulating your arousal levels brings your physical, mental, and emotional processes under control, thereby allowing you to perform at your best. If you are ready "mentally," it is most likely that you are ready "physically" as well. While competitive anxiety and tension cannot altogether be avoided, they can be managed with psychological strategies such as thought stopping, positive self-talk, energization, or relaxation.

Energization

I am sure you've experienced times when you weren't motivated to exercise. It could be that you were bored with training, there wasn't enough imminent competition, or because you were physically exhausted. If you notice that your lack of energy is indicative of a general pattern, then it's wise to take time away from training. One of the biggest mistakes you can make as a bodybuilder is to push through hard training without appropriate recovery

Table 10.1   Emotions Associated With Arousal

Optimal arousal	Overarousal	Underarousal
Calm	Nervous	Lethargic
Focused	Scattered	Bored
Energized	Hyper	Sluggish
Optimally challenged	Overly challenged	Not challenged
Mastery	Not enough mastery	Too much mastery
In control	Out of control	Overcontrolled
Confident	Not confident	Overconfident
Committed	Overcommitted	Undercommitted
"I can do it!"	"I have to do it!"	"Why bother?"

or rest. If you continue with this pattern it's likely you'll lose the desire to train, and it may even lead to injury. Take a week off and enjoy other sport and leisure activities. Go for a cycle through some wooded trails, play soccer with your children, or go to the swimming pool for a leisurely swim. When you go back to training be sure that you start out easy and continue to take "easy" weeks once you resume high-intensity training.

Sometimes you will just need a mental and physical "boost" to help you get through one or two workouts. Remember, most bodybuilders will function at their best if they can get into a high level of arousal. High arousal levels lead to better focus during the workout and enable you to train with greater intensity. The following techniques can be used to energize you and get you into that optimal state of arousal.

- Use imagery. You can imagine yourself as a ferocious bear or a pouncing tiger as you are about to complete a training set.
- Use suggestion. Convince yourself that you have lots of energy and that you can feel it flowing through you. Statements like " I can feel myself getting stronger during this workout," or " I can feel myself becoming more alert and focused" can be helpful. You are not crazy if you talk to yourself in the gym.
- Set challenges. Create a competitive environment for yourself by setting goals for each set. See if you can increase the weight between sets, decrease the rest interval between sets, or see how many times you can lift a lighter weight before you experience muscular fatigue.

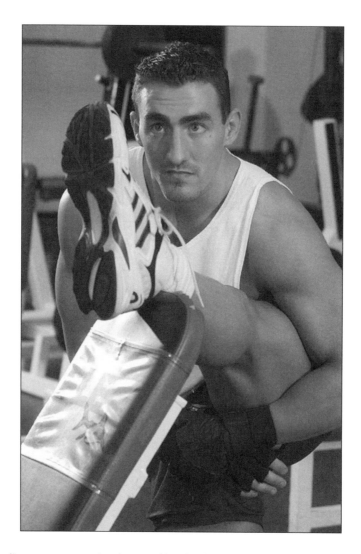

Understanding your own optimal arousal level will allow you to perform your best in every workout.

- Use music. Music can be extremely invigorating and can get you ready for the workout. Wear a headset with your own music if you do not like the music played in your gym.
- Warm up. The warm-up could be done at a faster pace than normal. Instead of casually riding the exercise bike before you workout, try a more intense ride with music of your choice.
- Add variety. Be prepared to change your workout to increase arousal levels. It is easy to get bored of workouts that never change. Workout programs should be adjusted at least every six weeks. You may even find that a visit to different gym is enough to increase your arousal levels and get you through the workout.

Relaxation

If your mind and body are relaxed, you will probably have an optimal training session. Relaxation can facilitate recovery between workouts and promote the onset of sleep. It may also relieve the muscular tension that produces headaches or lower back pain. As noted earlier in this book, relaxation is easy to learn and can enhance muscular development.

Relaxation is characterized by an absence of activity and tension. Relaxing the body involves the easing of muscle tension and the regulation of breathing. Relaxing the mind involves the easing of mental tension by blocking out negative thoughts. Understanding the mind-body connection is crucial to learning proper relaxation technique. A change in the mind almost always causes a corresponding change in the body. In other words, if your mind is relaxed, your body will also be relaxed.

Relaxation can be done at any time, and in any place, but it needs to be used in appropriate situations. Complete relaxation is particularly useful when you are tired, worried, or feeling stressed, but you should not use a complete relaxation exercise before or during a workout. Indeed, momentary relaxation is most appropriate for training and competition.

The amount of relaxation you need will depend on many factors, including your usual stress-management pattern, the presence of other bodybuilders, the relationship between you and your training partner, the time of year, the significance and level of the competition, and the size of the audience. Every bodybuilder will need to determine his or her own optimal level of arousal and the corresponding level of relaxation necessary to achieve an optimal performance.

The best way to determine this is to monitor your arousal level (i.e., heart and breathing rates, sweating, "butterflies," nervousness, and so on) before and during workouts. Ask yourself which workouts are your best. When are you completely relaxed, "pumped up," or somewhere between the two? When is your level of arousal low, moderate, or high?

You will also need to distinguish between complete and momentary relaxation. Both are important, but they play different roles in enhancing bodybuilding success. Complete relaxation involves gradually relaxing the major muscle groups to the point where each muscle group is fully relaxed. This can be accomplished using a number of different techniques including progressive relaxation. Complete relaxation would be appropriate when you have difficulty sleeping, are overly aroused, or are facing a particularly difficult competition.

Momentary relaxation is an extension of complete relaxation and is appropriate during a workout, show, or competition. Athletes who are capable of completely relaxing gain the most benefit from momentary relaxation. During a workout, there are times when you need to rechannel your energy and resources to finish the workout as strong as possible. Rechanneling energy is also necessary between difficult sets. In other words,

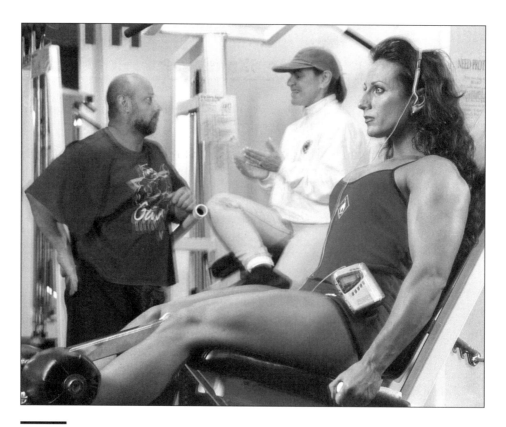

Relaxed awareness is key to effective training sessions.

use momentary relaxation whenever you feel that you are losing focus or becoming overly aroused. In this way, you can maintain "relaxed awareness," a state in which you are completely aware of what is going on and know what you must do to be successful but are functioning at your optimal level of arousal.

Relaxation Methods

Being aware of how you handle tense situations is the first step in relaxation training. Read over the questions in exercise 10.4 and think about the ways tension and anxiety affect your training and competition. Your responses will help you become more aware of how you currently handle tense situations. The next step is learning the methods of relaxation.

Note: Just like any other sport skill, relaxation skills must be practiced on a regular basis. While learning, it is best to practice relaxation techniques away from the gym. Once the skill is developed, you can introduce it at the gym, on the beach, and in the competitive arena. Most bodybuilders will notice some improvement in their ability to relax within two to three weeks. If you do not see any significant improvement, however, stick to your

Exercise 10.4 How Do You Handle Yourself In Anxious Situations?

Instructions: Read through each question below and answer in the space provided. Be sure to answer in complete sentences.

1. When you are lifting poorly in training or showing poorly in competition, do you start to feel out of control? Do you convince yourself that there is nothing you can do about the situation?

   _____

   _____

   _____

   _____

2. When your training partner gives you direct feedback or gets angry at you, do you use this information to improve or do you consider it a personal attack?

   _____

   _____

   _____

   _____

3. Do you let your training partner's poor training habits affect your development? Does it make you angry or even more determined to make sure that you train properly?

   _____

   _____

   _____

   _____

4. Are you aware of your stress level? Are you worried about your development? What about the antics of your training partner? Do you think these will affect your development?

   _____

   _____

   _____

   _____

When to Use Relaxation Strategies

Before Warming Up

Begin your warm-up with some form of relaxation to give you a clear sense of how you are feeling physically, mentally and emotionally. If you are feeling overaroused, you may want to continue the relaxation process longer so that you are in the optimal state of arousal. In general, if you are less experienced in bodybuilding and using relaxation, you should perform the relaxation technique just before your workout.

When Learning a New Skill

Learning a new skill, such as Olympic-style lifting, can be challenging, but too many practice sessions can lead to inefficient learning patterns and stagnation. Practice sessions should emphasize quality, not quantity. This also applies to your workouts: short, intense workouts are the most effective. By interspersing relaxation periods into your workouts you increase the "pump" in the working muscles.

While Warming Down

After a workout, you should do some simple relaxation exercises to help return you to a balanced physical state. This process can be quite stimulating and can also reduce the risk of injury associated with overuse.

Before Visualization

Use relaxation before any visualization exercise. This will not only enable you to focus more intently but also help you maximize the benefit from the visualization.

practice routine for several weeks. You will eventually see improvement. Developing relaxation skills takes time.

The following relaxation techniques are designed to either relax the mind or relax the body. Classified in three different categories—breathing exercises, progressive relaxation, and Benson's Relaxation Response—each of these methods can be used to achieve a state of relaxation that will enhance bodybuilding performance. The level of relaxation achieved, the time required to achieve a relaxed state, and the time to sufficiently learn the skill will vary depending on the method and the individual bodybuilder.

Breathing Exercises

Breathing properly is not only relaxing; it also facilitates lifting performance by increasing the amount of oxygen in the blood and promoting proper lifting technique. Unfortunately, most bodybuilders have never been taught the merits or techniques of proper breathing and therefore have developed ineffective breathing patterns. This is compounded under stressful conditions such as personal best lifts or while posing in an important competition, because the breathing patterns of most people become even more shallow under stress.

The good news is, learning to breathe properly is one of the easiest skills to learn. Learning to breathe in a deep, slow, controlled manner will facilitate a "relaxation response." A relaxation response is evidenced by decreased heart and breathing rates, lowered blood pressure, slower brain waves, and an overall reduction in the speed of metabolism. A relaxation response can be elicited to varying degrees depending on the individual bodybuilder.

How do you breathe? Try exercise 10.5 to see what kind of breathing you do. Read the steps first, then go back and perform them.

Exercise 10.5 | Breathing Exercise

1. Stand in front of a mirror, or ask a friend to observe you.

2. Place your left hand on your upper chest and place your right hand on your lower abdomen.

3. Take a big breath, then hold it for a slow count of three (1 Mississippi, 2 Mississippi, 3 Mississippi).

4. Slowly let it go, with your lips pursed, as if blowing on a spoonful of hot soup.

5. Repeat these steps again, this time paying attention to which hand is moving.

6. Which hand moved, your upper or lower hand? If your lower hand moves in and out as you breath, you are using your diaphragm, which means you are breathing properly. If your upper hand moves, you are taking shallow breaths. Shallow breathing does nothing to help you relax, it only makes you hyperventilate and feel increasingly lightheaded and cold.

Breathing Exercises

The following breathing techniques are adapted from *Applied Sport Psychology*.

EXERCISE 10.6 COMPLETE BREATHING

To breathe correctly is to breathe deeply and slowly from the diaphragm. The diaphragm is the thin muscle that separates the lungs from the abdominal cavity. When you inhale, the diaphragm moves down slightly and pushes the abdomen outward. This causes a partial vacuum in the lungs, which immediately fill with air from the bottom up. Complete breathing, also called "deep breathing," causes a relaxation response, which is characterized by a sense of calm.

Here is how you do complete breathing:

- Imagine your lungs being divided into three levels: lower, middle, and upper.
- When you start to inhale, focus on filling the lower level with air by pushing your diaphragm down and your abdomen out.
- As you continue inhaling, fill the middle level by expanding your chest and stretching your rib cage.
- Fill the upper level by further expanding your chest and shoulders slightly.
- Hold the inhalation for three to five seconds.
- Exhale slowly by pulling your abdomen in and lowering your chest and shoulders.
- Force all the air out of your lungs and let all your chest and abdomen relax.

The primary advantage of complete breathing is that you can achieve momentary relaxation with one breath. One or two breaths immediately before a set of squats or between sets of preacher curls will calm you. It does require some practice, but it is easy to learn.

EXERCISE 10.7 RHYTHMIC BREATHING

Rhythmic breathing is a slightly more sophisticated version of complete breathing, in that you coordinate your breathing pattern with a measured, rhythmic count. More relaxing than complete breathing, rhythmic breathing is an excellent technique to use between sets.

- Slowly inhale to the count of 4.
- Hold it to the count of 4.
- Slowly exhale to the count of 4.
- Hold the exhalation for the count of 4.

EXERCISE 10.8 RATIO BREATHING

More relaxing than rhythmic breathing, ratio breathing requires an inhale-exhale ratio of 1 to 2. That means, you count to 4 as you inhale but count to 8 when you exhale. This method requires a deep, full breath at the start and forces you to be more conscious about controlling your inhalation and exhalation. This is particularly helpful when you are about to complete the heaviest sets of an exercise, because it helps you to relax as well as focus your mental energy on the task at hand.

EXERCISE 10.9 CENTERING

Centering, a technique advocated by Bob Nideffer in his book *An Athlete's Guide to Mental Training*, is more than a breathing and relaxation technique. Centering is also a focusing technique.[3]

- Start out by sitting up straight in a firm chair.
- Consciously relax your neck and shoulder muscles, and open your mouth slightly.
- Ensuring that your abdomen is extending outward and that you are staying relaxed in your neck and shoulders, inhale slowly from the diaphragm. Do not allow your chest to expand or your shoulders to rise.
- Exhale slowly, focusing on the feelings in your abdomen. Notice the abdominals relaxing. As you exhale, let your knees relax, causing a feeling of heaviness, like you are anchored to the floor.
- Repeat the technique twice. (Three repetitions should be sufficient.) Eventually you will be able to center with one inhale and exhale.

According to Nideffer, centering can be beneficial in the following situations:

- Just before the start of a workout or competition
- Immediately before a "finite" performance, a performance that stands by itself (such as going for a personal best RM bench press)
- When you start to lose your focus or when you feel tired
- When you "must" perform perfectly
- During breaks in a workout or show, such as between sets or before and during your stage opportunity

Progressive Relaxation

The objective of progressive relaxation is to train the muscles to become sensitive to tension and then release that tension. Progressive relaxation is a consistent favorite among aesthetic sport athletes (dancers, figure skaters, synchronized swimmers, gymnasts, and bodybuilders) because it promotes the mind-body connection.

Bodybuilders who are already able to differentiate between efficient and inefficient muscular tension will have a distinct advantage in learning muscle-to-mind techniques. When powering their way through a difficult set of squats bodybuilders need to recruit every muscle fiber in their legs to get a maximum lift. Too often, however, inexperienced bodybuilders tense not only their legs but every muscle in their bodies, including the biceps or deltoids, muscles not involved in the lift. This renders an optimal set of squats impossible, because the biceps are providing inefficient muscle tension.

Like its name suggests, progressive relaxation consists of a progressive series of muscle contractions and relaxations, focusing on a specific muscle group at a time. Progressive relaxation is not only an excellent technique for controlling competitive anxiety; it is also helpful in falling asleep after a heavy workout or the night before an important competition. The progres-

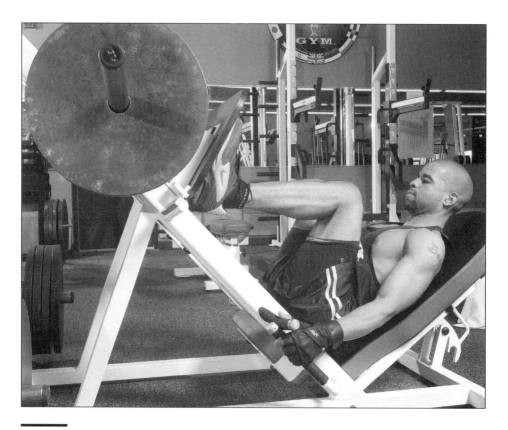

Learn to differentiate between efficient and inefficient muscular tension during your workout.

sion, in general, moves from the extremities (fingers and toes) to the central region (abdomen and chest).

Following is one variation of progressive relaxation that should be practiced on a regular basis before training, after training, or whenever you need to relax. You may want to record this on a tape so that you can do it alone. Once you feel more comfortable with the technique, you will be able to use the appropriate progression without having to be led through it.

1. Lie down in a comfortable position in a quiet environment. Loosen your clothing, remove your shoes, and let your body go limp.

2. Raise your left leg 6 inches off the floor and flex your toes back toward your head. Hold this flexed tension for 10 seconds. Saying, "Let go" to yourself, stop flexing. Let your leg fall back down. Let your left leg rest for 10 seconds and feel the tension flowing out of it. Feel the heaviness and warmth of your leg and foot. Repeat with the same leg.

   Repeat the exercise using your right leg and foot.

3. Lying down, tighten the thigh and buttock muscles of both legs as hard as you can for at least 10 seconds. Release the tension abruptly,

saying "Let go" to yourself. Feel the tension flowing out of these muscles. Relax for 10 seconds.

Repeat the exercise.

4. Tighten your abdominals, making them as hard as you can. Maintain this tension for 10 seconds. Relax these muscles and feel the tension flow out of them. Relax for 10 seconds.

Repeat the exercise.

5. Arch your back so that only your shoulders and buttocks are touching the floor. Feel the tension in the muscles along your back. Maintain this arch for 10 seconds. Let your back collapse back on the floor and completely relax. Feel the tension flow out.

Repeat the exercise.

6. Clench your right hand into a fist and increase the grip until you feel real tension throughout your hand and forearm. Hold this tension for 10 seconds. Slowly relax your hand, letting the tension flow out of the hand and forearm. Repeat with the same hand.

Repeat the exercise using your left hand and forearm.

7. Bend your right elbow and create tension in your right biceps. Tense it as hard as you can and hold it for 10 seconds. Relax and straighten the arm and allow the tension to flow out smoothly. Repeat with the same arm.

Repeat the exercise using your left arm.

8. Take a deep breath and hold it in your upper chest. At the same time, pull your shoulders back as though you were trying to touch your shoulder blades together. This should create a high level of tension across your chest, around your shoulders, and in your upper back. Hold this tension for 10 seconds. Slowly exhaling, let your shoulders relax. Relax for 10 seconds.

Repeat the exercise.

9. Press your head back against the mat or floor until you feel tension in your neck region. Hold that tension for 10 seconds and then relax by bringing your head back to a normal position.

Repeat the exercise.

10. Bring your head forward until it is resting on your chest. Create maximum tension in your throat and the back of your neck. Hold for 10 seconds, and then relax by bringing your head back to a normal position.

Repeat the exercise.

11. Wrinkle your forehead as hard as you can and hold it for 10 seconds. Relax by allowing your face and forehead to smooth out.

Repeat the exercise.

12. Closing your eyes, turn down the edges of your mouth into a deep frown. Feel the tension between your eyes and eyebrows. Hold for 10 seconds, and then relax your face and gently open your eyes.

   Repeat the exercise.

13. Squint your eyes tighter and tighter until you can feel the tension in your eyes. Hold for 10 seconds and then relax, gently and slowly opening your eyes.

   Repeat the exercise one more time.

14. Clench your jaw and bite down hard. Note the tension in your jaw. Hold this for 10 seconds, and then relax by parting your lips and letting your face become completely devoid of any expression.

   Repeat the exercise.

15. Purse your lips together, forming an "O". Feel the tension across your lips and cheeks. Hold for 10 seconds, and then relax by parting your lips slightly.

   Repeat the exercise.

Progressive relaxation requires considerable practice before mastery is achieved, so it is important to practice the exercises on a daily basis. Once you have learned to recognize muscle tension and relaxation, you can start to decrease the contractions for each muscle group until you no longer need to contract the muscles to achieve relaxation. Remember, the essence of progressive relaxation is learning how to recognize and consciously release muscular tension.

Benson's Relaxation Response

One of the most effective relaxation methods, Dr. Herbert Benson's Relaxation Response[4,5] can be mastered with just a few minutes of practice each day. It can be used not only before and after workouts but also during difficult training sessions. The Relaxation Response can be done at home, at school, in the car, or while riding the bus. A relaxed state can be achieved anywhere and at any time of day.

Changes produced by Benson's Relaxation Response can counteract the discomfort and pain of physical exertion. Research has shown that those who develop and regularly use Benson's Relaxation Response can also

- relieve headaches;
- reduce blood pressure and control hypertension;
- enhance creativity, especially when experiencing a block;
- overcome sleep disorders;
- prevent hyperventilation;
- alleviate backaches;

- control panic attacks;
- lower low-density cholesterol levels; and
- alleviate symptoms of anxiety, including nausea, vomiting, diarrhea, constipation, short temper, and the inability to get along with others.

For Benson's Relaxation Response to be effective while you are learning it, four basic elements must be present at all times. Once you have learned the technique, only two elements are necessary: focus object and passive attitude. In other words, you will no longer have to have a quiet environment or comfortable position to elicit the Relaxation Response.

1. Focus object: This object may be a word or sound, a symbol, a feeling—anything you choose. The purpose of having a focus object is to return to that object when you feel distracted.

2. Quiet: You must "turn off" not only mental distractions, but also distractions around you.

3. Passive attitude: Characterized by the absence of all negative thoughts and distractions, a passive attitude is the most essential factor in Benson's Relaxation Response. A passive attitude does not mean that you do not train hard or exert effort; it is simply a positive mental approach to relaxation.

4. Comfort: You should be comfortable enough to remain in the same position for at least 20 minutes without falling asleep. Usually a sitting position is recommended.

The following are Relaxation Response steps.

1.   Pick a word or brief phrase that reflects your personality or the sport of bodybuilding. This word will become your focal point throughout the Relaxation Response. Because meditation is an integral part of the Relaxation Response technique, it is important to pick a word, phrase, or object that holds special meaning for you. The more personal it is, the more deeply involved you will get in the technique. You will look forward to practicing it and you will do it more consistently.

When choosing an appropriate word or phrase, take a few things into consideration. First, the word or phrase must be easy to pronounce and remember. Second, the words should be short enough to say silently as you exhale a breath. Examples of some words you might consider: *one, out, in, strong, right, left, easy, power,* or *relax.*

2.   Choose a comfortable position. The position must be comfortable enough so that it can be maintained for relatively long periods of time, but uncomfortable enough that you will not fall asleep.

3.   Close your eyes. Avoid squinting or squeezing your eyes. Close them easily and naturally. The movement should be effortless.

4. Relax your muscles. Starting with your feet and progressing up to your calves, thighs, and abdomen, relax the various muscle groups in your body. (Use the progressive relaxation or body scan techniques discussed earlier in this chapter to help you.) Loosen up your head, neck, and shoulders by gently rolling your head around and shrugging your shoulders slightly. Stretch and then relax your arms and hands, allowing them to drape naturally onto your lap. Avoid grasping your knees or legs, crossing your arms, or clasping your hands tightly together.

5. Become aware of your breathing, and start to focus on your word or phrase. Breathe slowly and naturally, without forcing a rhythm. On each exhale, silently repeat the word or phrase you have chosen. If you are unable to think of a word or phrase to repeat, you can elicit the Relaxation Response without saying anything, instead focusing your awareness on the expansion of your abdomen as you inhale and the contraction as you exhale.

6. As you sit quietly, repeating your focus word or phrase, thoughts will inevitably begin to bombard your mind. You may see mental images or patterns that distract you. These lapses are natural. They happen to everyone. The key to dealing with these interruptions is learning to respond to them in a casual, passive way. Do not force the interruptions out of your mind. Simply say "oh well," and begin to think about your focus word or object again. Likewise, if you are distracted by an itch or uncomfortable clothing, go ahead and take care of the distraction: scratch, or remove the clothing as you continue focusing on your word or phrase.

Do not be discouraged if the distracting thoughts occur the entire time you're meditating; they're natural. With regular practice, you will learn to disregard the distractions that push their way into your consciousness— including the nagging doubts about how well you are performing the technique and whether it is working.

7. Practice the technique for 10 to 20 minutes at the most, but do not time the sessions. The sound of an alarm would startle you, or cause you to anticipate the signal. Instead, keep a watch or clock in plain sight, and sneak a peek when you think about the time. If the practice time has not passed, close your eyes again and return to your focus word or phrase until the full time has elapsed.

Once the session is over, sit quietly and keep your eyes closed for a full minute or two. Stop repeating your focus word or phrase. Allow regular thoughts to enter your mind once again. Finally, open your eyes slowly and sit quietly for another full minute or two. If you stand up immediately, you may feel dizzy. This is not dangerous, but it is unnecessary.

8. Practice the technique twice a day. Just as it takes a lot of practice to develop physical skills, it also takes practice to effectively elicit relaxation. Most people practice before breakfast and before dinner. The exact time you schedule your sessions is up to you, but the method seems to work best on an empty stomach.

Once you feel comfortable with it, you can begin to use the Relaxation Response technique before, during, and after workouts and competitions. Here are some tips for using the Relaxation Response specifically in the sport of bodybuilding.

- Do your usual stretching and warm-up exercises before you begin using the Relaxation Response.
- During your warm-up in the locker room or while riding a bike, close your eyes to avoid distractions. If you are using the Relaxation Response between sets or during a rest period, keep your eyes open so that you can maintain focus on the activity at the same time.
- Become aware of your breathing. After you fall into a regular pattern, focus on the rhythm of your breathing. As you exhale, say your focus word or phrase silently. Choose a word that represents the quality you would like to portray during your next set. For example, if you want to be powerful as you rip through another set of bench presses, you might choose the word *power*. If you want to maintain control, you might use *control*.
- When you have completed your workout, return to your normal post-workout routine. This helps you to break away from your "relaxed awareness" mode.

To improve your ability to relax and to effectively use relaxation as a performance tool, you must practice consistently and often. Make sure that you practice the breathing exercises and both the progressive relaxation and Relaxation Response techniques so that you will have three methods to choose from. Where you choose to practice is unimportant, as long as you practice regularly. You should notice some improvement within two to three weeks of regular practice. Exercise 10.10 will show you how to record your relaxation levels before and after relaxation techniques.

Focus

One of the most important skills you will develop is the ability to focus your attention without being distracted. One of the most common problems for young athletes is their inability to focus when they most need to, namely, under pressure. You have probably seen what happens when bodybuilders lose their focus: their perception is hampered, they make poor exercise choices, they lack adequate intensity for muscle growth, they take too many water breaks, they rest too long between sets, and they spend too much time looking around the weight room for ideas of what to do next. At the very least, their workouts are ineffective and overly long. At the extreme, their workouts are unsafe, for themselves and those around them.

What do you think about when someone tells you to concentrate? When your training partner tells you to concentrate, are you confused about

Exercise 10.10 | Relaxation Practice Evaluation

Instructions: Use the chart below to record your use of relaxation techniques. Use the following scale for the ratings in the last two columns: 1 = very tense, 2 = tense, 3 = normal, 4 = relaxed, 5 = completely.

Relaxation Practice Evaluation

Date	Method rating	Time of day	Duration	Rating (before)	Rating (after)

exactly what he or she wants you to do? Do you ever tell yourself to concentrate and then just continue lifting with the same preoccupied mindset?

The ability to concentrate in the weight room or under pressure at competitions is difficult to develop. Many bodybuilders stare out in space, scrunch up their foreheads, and tighten their jaws, all in attempt to look like they are concentrating. More than likely, they are so focused on concentrating that they are no longer concentrating on the workout. Focus requires considerable practice, instruction, and experience. Understanding exactly how to focus your attention and concentrate on the task at hand will go a long way in improving your mental toughness and development.

As you probably know, the bodybuilding environment can be tremendously distracting. Busy gyms, poor equipment, other muscular bodies, and loud music—external stimuli can overpower even the most serious attempts at focusing. But did you know that bodybuilders can also be distracted by internal stimuli, such as worrying about their inadequacies, thinking about things unrelated to their performance, and simply thinking too much? Unless you are able to totally focus on your workout, you will not perform as well as you could. Consistent lack of focus can impede long-term development.

As a bodybuilder, recreational or serious, you must learn to increase your selective awareness, that is, awareness of task-relevant stimuli with a corresponding lack of awareness of irrelevant and distracting stimuli. In bodybuilding, relevant stimuli would include the feel of an exercise, the familiarity of gym equipment, and the encouraging words from your training partner. Irrelevant stimuli would include other bodybuilders, lights in the gym, and even music if you found that it did not motivate you toward your goal of muscular development.

Types of Focus

Are you the type of person who likes to work on one project at a time and see it to completion before starting another project? Or do you prefer working on many things at the same time, and if so, are you able to get all your projects completed? Different people focus their attention differently, whether at school, work, or play. Bodybuilders are no different.

In bodybuilding, you will need to control two characteristics of focusing: width and direction. First, you will need to establish the appropriate width of focus for your task, either broadening your focus to include many things at the same time or narrowing your focus to one specific thought or action. Before starting a chest workout, you will need a broad focus, one in which you are sensitive to the many different pieces of equipment designed to target the chest muscles. When you are ready to begin the workout, however, you will need to narrow your focus to the exercise itself, concentrating on the

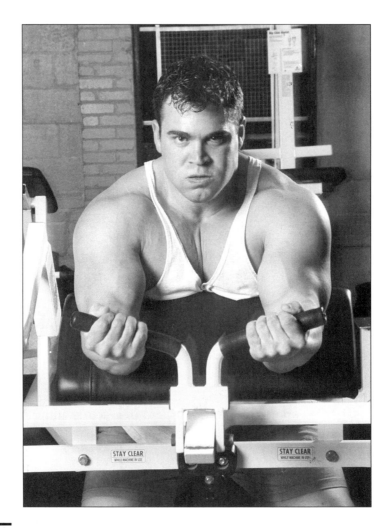

Concentration and focus are vital to achieving maximum results from your workout.

mechanics that will produce the muscle development and body shaping you desire. When you begin the set, you will need to further narrow your focus on the exercise for as long as one minute of "muscle blowing" intensity.

Second, you will need to control the direction of your focus. In some situations, you will need to focus internally, concentrating on your feelings, thoughts, and actions. In other situations, you will need to focus externally, concentrating on things other than yourself, such as the equipment or weight. Figure 10.2 illustrates the focusing characteristics required in four different bodybuilding situations.

As a bodybuilder, you find some characteristics of focusing more important than others. You will also find that these characteristics change, depending on the situation you find yourself in. For example, you will need a broad-

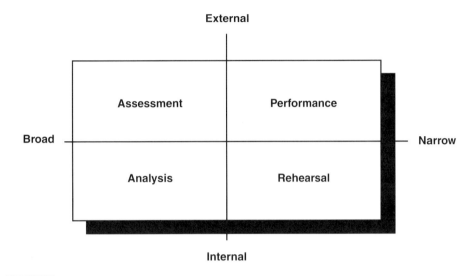

Figure 10.2   Types of focus.

internal focus to plan your workout after you have surveyed the weight room, but you need a broad-external focus to conduct the assessment of the equipment that is available to you. The narrow-internal focus of attention is one of visualization and mental rehearsal, in which you visualize yourself completing the set in a powerful way. The narrow-external focus, on the other hand, is the most helpful during a set, when you must maintain the most intense focus to complete your reps, particularly those final few that are often the most difficult.

During a workout, you will likely need to shift your focus many times, as described in Joanne's story below.

Joanne is a serious bodybuilder and fitness participant. When she enters the gym, Joanne looks over the number of people using the equipment (broad-external) and begins to mentally plan her workout (broad-internal). She goes into the locker room and begins to mentally prepare (narrow-internal) for the upcoming 45 minutes of muscle-building chest exercises. After the warm-up (conducted primarily in the broad-external focus), she sits down on the incline bench and thinks about the intensity required to maximize the exercise to its muscle-building potential (narrow-internal). She lies back on the bench, grips the bar, and lifts it off the rack with her eyes and mind focused on the bar (narrow-external). With increasing intensity, she rips off one rep after another while remaining focused on completing her goal (narrow-external). Completing the set and feeling exhausted, Joanne places the bar back on the rack and goes over the set in her mind (narrow-internal).

Profile in Strength: Carol Semple-Marzetta

Carol Semple-Marzetta could easily be called the "original queen" of fitness competitions. Since beginning her competitive career in 1991, she has revolutionalized the sport with her breathtaking feats of strength and flexibility. She has also won every major title in existence, including Ms. Fitness U.S.A., Ms. Fitness World, the Fitness International, and the Fitness Olympia. Now retired from professional fitness competitions, Carol currently works as a choreographer and personal trainer to fitness competitors. Currently completing her bachelor's degree in nutrition and exercise science, Carol serves as a role model to women of all fitness levels.

Mind to Muscle Principles:

1. Continually challenge yourself to achieve. Do not be satisfied with "good enough" when you want to be "great." Despite unparalleled success, Carol continually set the bar higher for herself. She says, "I absolutely loved competition. I got such satisfaction from setting a goal, training to achieve it, and then laying my cards on the table." Carol is well known for her meticulous preparation for competition, including hours of intense training, choreography, and practice of routines. Not surprisingly, she also became known for "blowing away the competition" with her spectacular fitness routines. "I prepared myself to compete against another Carol Semple-Marzetta. I trained like I was going to compete against myself."

2. Value your body for its health, strength, and flexibility rather than appearance only. Carol describes her approach to fitness as "all-cause morbidity." She says, "I'm dedicated to keeping my body healthy and strong so that I have more years of being active and mobile. Taking care of yourself now helps keep your quality of life as you age." Rather than obsess about her appearance, Carol takes care of her body with an eye toward the future. She understands the relationship between present lifestyle choices and long-term quality of life.

3. Become a role model and share your enthusiasm for strength training with other women. In her work as a personal trainer, Carol educates women about building muscle and the importance of healthy nutrition. "For me," she says, "that's what bodybuilding is about—empowering other women to become strong." Carol hopes to use her education to educate women in the future: "I would like to continue speaking publicly, personal training, and preparing fitness competitors. That's my way of passing it on."

Focusing Exercises

As with any mental skill, the ability to focus is a learned skill that can be improved. First, your level of arousal can play a critical role in your ability to focus. Increases in your level of arousal may narrow the width and direction of your focus. For example, overarousal may produce a narrow-internal focus while underarousal may cause a broad-external focus. It's for this reason that getting into the optimal zone of arousal is so critical. Second, you can practice your focusing skills with a number of different mental exercises. Read through each of the focusing exercises on the following pages (exercises 10.11 to 10.17) and then decide on two or three to try. With regular practice, you will see dramatic improvements in your ability to focus during training and competition.

EXERCISE 10.11 EXPANDING AWARENESS

This exercise, originally developed by Gauron,[6] is designed to help bodybuilders experience different characteristics of focusing. Moving from a narrow focus to a broad focus gives you a deeper appreciation for the different types of focus. As you practice, you develop the ability to adjust your focus during workouts. Then you can train with focus and intensity.

1. Breathe normally and think about your breathing. For the next minute, begin to breathe more deeply and slowly from your diaphragm while keeping your shoulders, chest, and neck relaxed. Alternate between normal and deep breathing, performing three or four normal breaths and then three or four deep breaths, until your deep breathing is regular and relaxed.

2. Begin to pay attention to what you hear by first identifying each sound and then mentally labeling it: footsteps, a crying baby, adult voices, and so on. Now try to listen to all the sounds at once, without identifying any particular sound. The sounds should begin to blend together.

3. Become aware of physical sensations, such as feeling your weight being supported as you sit. Before moving on to a different sensation, label the one you are currently experiencing, considering both its quality and its source. For example, you could say that your supported weight is feeling "heavy" and "compact." As you did with the sounds, begin to blend all of the physical sensations you are feeling, to the point where you are unable to identify any particular sensation.

4. Focus on your thoughts and emotions. Let each thought or emotion enter your consciousness, then label it and identify its source. Remain calm, no matter what the quality of the thought or emotion. Notice another one, and another, then let all of your thoughts and emotions blend together.

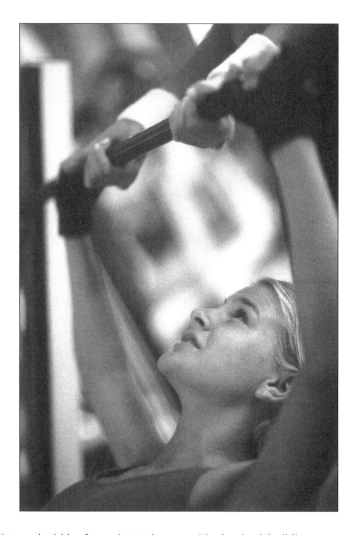

The direction and width of your intensity are critical to bodybuilding success.

5. Open your eyes and visually focus on an object ahead of you. While you are looking ahead, try to take in as much of the room as possible. Notice what you see on the walls, the type of furniture, and so on. Now begin to focus on the object ahead of you again, narrowing your focus until it is the only object you see. Imagine you are looking through a tunnel to the object at the other end. Now begin to broaden your focus again, until you can see everything in the room.

EXERCISE 10.12 QUICK SHIFT AND FIND EXERCISE

This exercise is an excellent drill to learn to change your focus quickly. This exercise can be done anywhere at the gym—while sitting on an exercise bike or in the nutritional supplement area. This exercise can also be effective when watching other bodybuilders.

1. On a piece of paper, list the exercise equipment you most like to use. Narrow your focus to the first piece of equipment on your list. Do not take your eyes off it for 15 to 20 seconds.

2. Now look around the gym, find that same piece of equipment, and narrow your focus onto it. Notice how the equipment is being used and imagine yourself using the equipment in a high-intensity workout.

3. Alternate between the list of equipment and the piece of equipment in the gym. Try to focus for different time intervals. For example, you may start out by focusing for 3 to 5 seconds on the list and then switch to the piece of equipment for another 3 to 5 seconds. Gradually increase the time interval to as much as 15 to 20 seconds

Try to make this exercise fun by adding variety to your focusing practice. For example, focus on one bodybuilder in the gym (narrow-external), then switch to seeing everyone in the gym (broad-external), and then go back to focusing on the one bodybuilder (narrow-external).

EXERCISE 10.13 HUB EXPANSION EXERCISE

This exercise is best done sitting down at a desk with a partner. Draw a hub on a piece of paper, similar to the one shown in figure 10.3. In the circle,

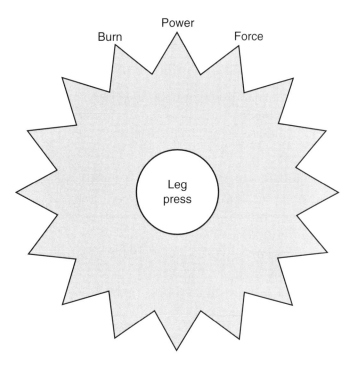

Figure 10.3 Hub expansion.

write the term *leg press* (or the name of any piece of equipment or bodybuilding concept). This is your narrow focus concept.

1. Begin by focusing on *leg press* (or other narrow focus concept) at the center of the hub.

2. Have your partner say "expand." At this point, broaden your focus and write down the first word that comes to your mind. The word you write should relate to your narrow focus concept.

3. After approximately five seconds, return your focus back to your narrow focus concept.

4. Continue to narrow and broaden your focus until all of the points at the outer edge of the hub are labeled. If you have difficulty coming up with words for the outer edge of the hub, this is a good indication that you are good at narrowing your focus but struggle to broaden your focus quickly.

EXERCISE 10.14 CONCENTRATED FOCUS EXERCISE

Sit quietly, close your eyes, and see how long you can focus on a single thought. Start out by trying to focus on the same thought for 10 seconds, then 20 seconds, then 30 seconds, and so on. You can also try this exercise visually. Concentrate on a picture of a bodybuilder or workout scene.

Practice on extending your focusing ability for 5 to 10 minutes each day. If distracting thoughts enter your mind, bring your attention back to your thought or picture. Do not shut out the thoughts or feelings. Just gently regain your focus.

EXERCISE 10.15 SHUTTLING

This exercise was created by Dr. John Hogg (1995).[7] It's designed to help you develop your internal and external focusing skills. It's good practice for the gym environment in which you must first analyze, then execute, an exercise.

1. Sit comfortably in a quiet place and close your eyes.

2. Tune in to some sensation, thought, or feeling that you are experiencing and say to yourself, "Now I am aware of feeling (the thought, feeling, or sensation)."

3. Open your eyes and say to yourself, "Now I am aware of (something that is happening outside of yourself)."

4. Repeat this process for a few minutes, shifting from an internal focus to an external focus, and back again.

EXERCISE 10.16 NARROWING GRID EXERCISE

The focus grid shown in figure 10.4 is an excellent tool for developing the skill of focus narrowing. Scattered randomly throughout the grid are 100 numbers, ranging from 00 to 99. Starting with 00, find each number in

84	27	51	78	59	52	13	85	61	55
28	60	92	04	97	90	31	57	29	33
32	96	65	39	80	77	49	86	18	70
76	87	71	95	98	81	01	46	88	00
48	82	89	47	35	17	10	42	62	34
44	67	93	11	07	43	72	94	69	56
53	79	05	22	54	74	58	14	91	02
06	68	99	75	26	15	41	66	20	40
50	09	64	08	38	30	36	45	83	24
03	73	21	23	16	37	25	19	12	63

Figure 10.4   Focus grid.

numerical order. For example, after 00 you need to look for 01, then 02, then 03, and so on. When you find each number, cross it out and move on to the next number. See how many you can find in one minute. If you can identify 30 or more in sequence within one minute, your focus-narrowing ability is good.

You can add variety to this exercise by starting with a different number and working in the opposite direction. For example, start at 99 and work backward. You can also challenge yourself by playing loud music, listening to the radio, or having someone talk to you while you are working through the focus grid. The better you are able to narrow your focus while being distracted, the better you will be able to narrow your focus during training and competition.

EXERCISE 10.17 FOCUS SWITCHING EXERCISE

For this exercise, which has been adapted from *Mental Skills for Swim Coaches* [8], you will need two radios. It also might help you to use a focus cue each time you focus. In other words, you may focus on a persons, voice or a musical instrument as you listen to the radios.

1. Place the radios about 20 feet apart, and tune each radio to a different station, adjusting them to the same volume. Use one radio as the signal, or stimulus, and the other as the noise, or distraction.

2. Stand equidistant between the radios.

3. Gradually focus on the signal, blocking out the noise. Take your time. Note how you are able to focus solely on the signal.

4. Now gradually switch your focus to the noise, blocking out the signal. Again, take your time. Note how you are able to focus only on the noise.

5. Try switching your focus from the signal to the noise, and back again, a couple of times. Be patient. Practice will help you shift your attention and become more selectively aware.

Once you are proficient at this skill, you can make the exercise a little more difficult by tuning in to two talk-radio programs. Again, determine which radio will be the signal and which will be the noise.

1. Gradually focus only on the signal. At the same time, notice how you are feeling. Does it give you a headache? Are you confused by the two sounds? Are you frustrated by this exercise? Go back now and repeat what you heard from the signal.

2. Now bring your focus to the noise. Again, monitor your mental processes and repeat what you hear on the noise radio. Persevere with the exercise until you can shift your attention with ease.

Focusing Guidelines for Bodybuilders

As you practice these focusing exercises and apply your newfound skills to your workouts and competitions, keep in mind the following guidelines for athletes, suggested by Hogg.[9]

- Be aware of the different focus demands of each skill, task, or situation. Identify what you must focus on at the gym and in competitions.

- Learn to increase your selective awareness.

- Anxiety about tough competition may cause you to narrow your focus too much, even to the point of losing control and sacrificing your strategy. You need to view competition in the proper light. It's only a competition and does not determine your failure or success as a person.

- Become aware of your preferred focus style. Do you naturally focus narrowly or broadly? Are you the kind of person that likes to do many tasks at the same time or just focus intently on one task at a time? Do you excel at sports where you mostly have to narrow (i.e., weight lifting, golf, rifle shooting, billiards) or do you excel at broadening sports (i.e., basketball, hockey, football)? Learn to condition yourself to using appropriate responses during quality training.

- If you think too much about the end result of a good workout (such as body shape or size), you could lose your focus. Instead keep your focus on the present moment and the process of exercising.

- To get a handle on all of the potential distractions you will face, practice your focus skills in a variety of different settings.
- Remember that elite performers are generally focused, that is, they are disturbed by neither internal nor external stimuli.
- Try not to let the avoidance of distractions become a distraction in itself. Try to adopt a more passive approach and let each distraction pass as it comes up.

As it is for most people, your thoughts and feelings will probably vary from day to day, in all likelihood, more than your physical sensations will. When you arrive at the gym for a workout, you will bring these thoughts and feelings with you, based on your experiences that day or week. These experiences may be negative, such as receiving a poor grade in school, breaking up with a girlfriend or boyfriend, having a fight with a loved one, or losing a job. They may also be positive, such as passing a difficult exam, being promoted, forming a new friendship, or getting tickets for an upcoming event. Whether your thoughts and feelings are positive or negative, they can be distracting and drain your energy.

The key to achieving your optimal workout is recognizing where your attention is focused. If your focus has nothing to do with bodybuilding, you will have to make the necessary adjustments. The easiest way to do this is to sit down, take a deep breath, and let your distracting thoughts pass. Acknowledge each one and then place it in the background so that you can focus on developing your body.

This has been formalized with a technique called Black Box Visualization in *Sporting Body Sporting Mind*. Black Box Visualization allows you to participate fully in your workout now by making a promise to deal with thoughts, feelings, worries, concerns, or whatever is distracting you from your workout at a more appropriate time, in this case, after your training. Initially, your Black Box Visualization should be led by a coach, training partner, or friend. Once you become familiar with the technique, you will be able to apply it on your own without outside guidance.

Although at first Black Box Visualization may seem overly simplistic, the more you practice the technique and use it before workouts and competitions, the more you will see its benefits. Over and over again, athletes claim that Black Box Visualization has significantly improved their ability to deal with distractions, internal and external. Indeed, every athlete I have coached, including bodybuilders, has found Black Box Visualization extremely helpful.

There is such a strong connection between your mind and body as you exercise that it becomes quite obvious that mental skills development is important. This is certainly the case with body awareness, arousal regulation, and focusing. Optimal performance in the gym, on the stage, and in life will come in those moments when your physical and mental dimensions are unified and equally developed. This book has provided you with a thorough

Black Box Visualization

Sit quietly, close your eyes, take a deep breath, and allow yourself to settle heavily into your chair as you breathe out slowly.

Imagine yourself sitting at a desk in front of a window. Look out and notice what you see, what the weather is like, what movement there may be. Then look down at the desk and notice a blank sheet of paper and a pen. Pick up the pen and write down whatever is worrying or exciting you, anything you identify as a distraction. As you write, see the shape of your handwriting on the page, hear the point of your pen slide over the paper, feel the weight of your upper body on your arm. If you find it easier, you can draw a picture to represent the distraction. When you have finished, put the pen down, fold up the piece of paper, and turn around. You see a box behind you. It may be on a shelf or on the floor. Notice how large it is and whether it is in the light or the shadow. Open the lid and put the folded piece of paper inside the box. Close the lid and turn back to the desk, settling back into your chair and once more looking out the window.

Open your eyes. You are ready to interact with those around you. Once your training session is over, again close your eyes and go back to this imaginary desk. Turn around, open the box, unfold the piece of paper, and look to see what you wrote or drew. Sometimes this will no longer be of interest. That's fine, but if the exercise is to continue to work—and with time it can become increasingly effective—the part of you that has been promised attention later must learn to trust that it will get that attention.

Adapted from Syer and Connolly 1984.[10]

understanding of the mental skills that are critical for bodybuilders. It has also suggested a number of different strategies and exercises that can help you to acquire and develop those mental skills. The next chapter is written specifically to those bodybuilders that desire to show off their hard-earned muscles in fitness and bodybuilding competitions.

CHAPTER 11

Peaking for Competition

Since 1965, the number of bodybuilding competitions has increased exponentially. Indeed, today there are regional, amateur, natural, and professional competitions too numerous to count. More recently, the number of fitness competitions has also blossomed over the past 10 to 15 years, to the point that they now have taken over female bodybuilding as the prime avenue of competition for women interested in muscle development and body shaping.

There are enough different bodybuilding and fitness competitions that anyone who wants to show off his or her hard work in the gym can do so. Just like running a road race, it's not necessary to win in order to enjoy and benefit from competition. The competition experience provides an additional incentive to stay focused on your training.

Preparing for a bodybuilding competition is difficult, to be sure. Not only must bodybuilders train for many years, but they must also commit to a 12- to 16-week marathon of fine-tuning the body for competition. This fine-tuning is a combination of the physiologically opposed tasks of maintaining a large quantity of muscle mass while shedding a large percentage of body fat.

This grueling cutting-up period requires discipline and determination 24 hours a day. Bodybuilders must pay meticulous attention to their diet, undergo intense weight-training sessions and countless hours of cardiovascular exercise, learn and practice mandatory poses and posing routines, all while attending to their everyday life activities such as a full-time job or school. It is not surprising, then, that a bodybuilder's mental state plays a critical role in this process. Indeed, many bodybuilders "lose their heads" and withdraw several weeks before the competition.

This chapter applies the many concepts discussed throughout this book to the competitive environment. It is designed to successfully guide you through the mental processes of competition, from the moment you commit to competing, to the moment you step off the stage.

Characteristics of Elite Athletes

"Athletes are not made; they are born." While this saying is not entirely true, it is clear that certain characteristics found among elite athletes are not found in less successful athletes. Knowing what these characteristics are will give you an idea of what it is going to take to be a successful, competitive bodybuilder. If you want to get more than the participation ribbon for your involvement in a competition, you may need some of the following attributes.

Competitiveness

Clearly, all athletes want to improve their skills. But improving is often not enough. Elite athletes understand that, while winning is an important part of the sport experience, the quality of personal performance is most important. They understand that they have little control over their opponents, and thus seek to control their own development.

Maybe you have never heard about the bodybuilder, Willie "I Need to Win" Wilson, that determined, after a disappointing finish, to come back and win the "Mr. Out of this World" bodybuilding competition the following year. For one full year, he religiously followed a carefully planned nutrition and supplement program, trained with an unheard of level of intensity, got the optimal amount of rest and sleep, and perfected a posing routine. By the time the competition rolled around he was bigger, stronger, and more ripped than he had ever been before. At the end of the competition, feeling confident that his new physique would earn him the first prize, he was naturally dejected to find out that he had finished in the exact same place as the year before. How could this be? What about all the improvements he had made? What happened was that at the same time that Willie "I Need to Win" Wilson was making significant improvements in his physique so was everybody else. He forgot that while it is important to be highly competitive that the "real" competition was against himself and not against others. The point is that you should desire to win every competition that you enter but more importantly is to enter every competition in better shape than the previous. Continually improving your body will increase the *likelihood* that you will beat others but you must remember that your improvement is no guarantee that you will.

Self-Efficacy

Successful bodybuilders know and understand what it takes to be the very best. They also know that they are capable of performing at their very best and getting considerable attention from judges, fans, and spectators. They are confident that they can create a championship body and that their body deserves to be appreciated by others. It is not that they are conceited or out of touch with reality; it is that they are highly confident in their ability to create a great body that will be recognized as one of the best. They simply have high self-efficacy.

Self-efficacy, a situationally specific form of self-confidence, is the belief that one is capable of performing the skills required to produce a certain

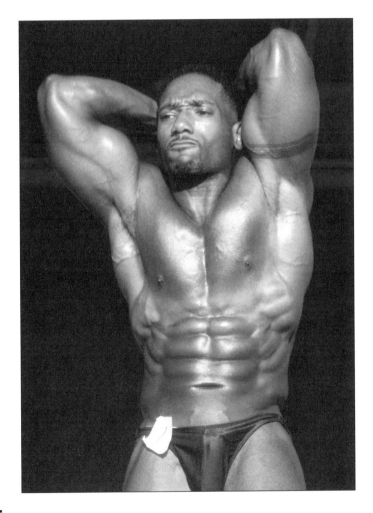

Believing in yourself and knowing that you are capable of excellence will lead to great performances.

outcome. On the capability front, you would have to believe yourself capable of committing to a regular program of weight training, training with high intensity workout after workout, and sticking with an appropriate muscle-building diet. Of course, being willing to commit to the bodybuilding lifestyle for the number of years necessary is also a factor. On the outcome side, you would have to believe that your developed muscular physique will be competitive.

Bodybuilders with high self-efficacy are highly motivated to train, eat low-fat diets, get adequate sleep, and make necessary adjustments to their lifestyle. Once they have created their optimal body, they are motivated to show it off because they know that it is going to be appreciated by judges and spectators alike.

Sensory Overload

Elite bodybuilders enjoy every aspect of competition. The lights, the roar of the crowd, the music, the rush of optimal performance, the fatigue after an optimal performance, the voice of the master of ceremonies—every sense is involved in the experience. While unnerving for most, the sensory overload on a bodybuilding stage is exhilarating and exciting for elite bodybuilders.

How do you get to the point where you find unnerving sensory overload to be exhilarating and exciting? As a competitive bodybuilder, the first step is to immerse yourself into many anxiety-producing situations. This forces an overload of your sensory system, helps you to develop appropriate physiological and psychological reactions to stressful situations, and gives you experience at maintaining control that can be utilized at competitions.

Certainly everyone can find some situation that elicits fear and anxiety. These are natural human reactions. Force yourself to speak in public, overcome your fear of snakes or spiders, wear your competition suit on a public beach. The better you become at controlling your response to anxiety, the better equipped you will be to control your anxiety at a competition.

Willingness to Take Risks

Competitive bodybuilders put their bodies on the line for all to see. Talk about risk taking! Is there any other sport in the world where there is a greater risk of damage to your body image and self-confidence? Is there any other sport where you have to display your half-naked body in front of hundreds or thousands of spectators and a panel of judges, and in which success is determined entirely by the look of your body? Of course, along with that risk come the thrill and excitement of showing off your hard work, not to mention the anticipation of the win.

If you want to be successful, you will have to learn to take calculated risks in training, nutrition, shedding body fat, and stage presentation. I am talking not about being stupid in your decisions but about being willing to try new training techniques and energy-rich foods, different cutting methods, and unique choreographed routines to get the attention of the judges and crowd. Sure, it may backfire, but only those bodybuilders who are prepared to risk will rise above the pack and become elite.

Reboundability

If sport were easy, everyone would be a champion athlete. The fact is, no sport is easy. Even the best of the best have setbacks and defeats. While disappointing, setbacks are a necessary part of sport. If nothing else, they make the victories and successes that much more enjoyable. In bodybuilding, a setback could be a significant injury, a new job that reduces your training time, the loss of your training partner, the closing down of your favorite gym, inadequate rest and shedding of body fat before a competition, or a poor performance. Any one of these setbacks can impinge on your muscular growth and self-esteem. The only guarantees in bodybuilding: (1) setbacks will happen, and (2) only you can determine how they will affect you.

The ability to take control of the situation is what reboundability is all about. Rebounding from a setback is the sign of a true champion. Elite athletes use setbacks to their advantage in two ways. First, they learn as much as possible about the cause of the setback, including how it might deter further development and the ways to prevent it from happening again. Second, elite athletes understand that they have an advantage over those athletes who are incapable of overcoming setbacks. So, if you want to be an elite bodybuilder, expect that you will have setbacks and learn to rebound from them more quickly than anyone else.

Ability to Get Into "The Zone"

Bodybuilding competitions can be stressful, and every bodybuilder responds to that stress differently. Elite bodybuilders understand that it is impossible to show their best if they are too relaxed before and during a competition. Mental sharpness is lost in a state of underarousal, making the chance of mental errors that much greater. Conversely, being too "pumped up," a state of overarousal, can lead to anxiety, distraction, and overwhelming worry and doubt. Elite bodybuilders try to reach an optimal state of arousal, otherwise known as "the zone," a perfect balance of stress and relaxation where they will function at their very best.

Take time to figure out what your state of optimal arousal is and how you reach it. For example, try to recall how you were feeling before your best and worst competitions. Did you prepare any differently? Was your confidence level higher or lower before those competitions? To be competitive, you will need to know what your state of optimal arousal is and be able to get yourself into "the zone" every time.

Mentally Preparing for Competition

No matter what the sport, every athlete must learn to prepare for competitions and events in a way that optimal performances will be realized more often than not. In bodybuilding, competitions are thought of as achievement contests in which the body, the product of a bodybuilder's hard work, is evaluated by neutral judges. The problem is that too many bodybuilders see competitions as a contest against another person rather a contest against themselves. For many bodybuilders, this creates a fear of failure, which renders them helpless against the natural stressors of competing on stage.

Fear of failure increases anxiety, interferes with realistic thinking, and increases the likelihood of "choking" while on stage. It also increases the risk of injury while warming up before a competition. Indeed, fear of failure

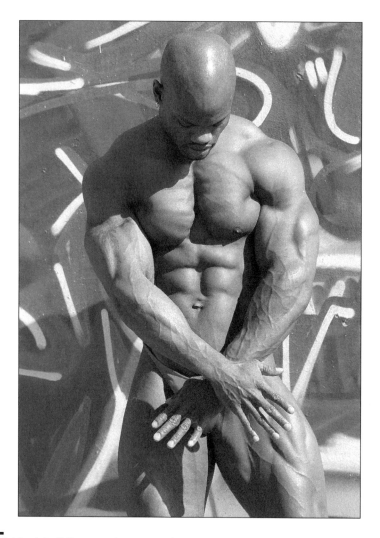

Successful bodybuilding requires you to be mentally prepared to show off your physical attributes.

promotes tentative and tenuous behavior, which can be harmful to a body-builder while lifting. Someone who fears failure is afraid of making a mistake in their training or nutritional program. They seek out the "sure" methods rather than attempt something that is a little newer but may produce significant positive changes. Ultimately, fear of failure takes away from the enjoyment of bodybuilding and leads many bodybuilders to drop out of the sport altogether. To overcome fear of failure, it is critical that you begin to view each competition as a learning experience, a source of unbiased information about your body.

Even if you overcome your fear of failure and compete against yourself, however, there is no guarantee of success. Indeed, having the best and fittest body is not even a guarantee of winning the prize. Some people always seem to win and others always seem to lose. Some athletes simply compete better than others. Maybe you are one of those people who can overcome your body weaknesses by outperforming those with better bodies. Maybe it is just the opposite for you. Understanding and developing the elements of competitive preparation will go a long way to ensuring your competitive success.

By reading this book, you have already developed a number of mental skills that could assist you in the competitive arena. If you want to be mentally prepared to compete, it is a good idea to periodically evaluate these skills, assessing how your practice is going and where you need to improve. Every three to four months, go through the checklist in exercise 11.1, adapted from Mark Anshel's *Sport Psychology*[1], to assess your progress in developing the mental and physical skills that maximize performance.

Weeks Before the Competition

After you have committed yourself to competing, there are a number of strategies you can use to ensure that you are at your best the day of the competition. The following strategies not only will help you perform your best, but they can also increase your enjoyment of the pre-competition phase. The pre-competitive phase is the final 12 weeks prior to the competition. It includes the final 4-6 weeks of the muscle building period and a 6- to 8-week cutting-up period. (For a detailed look at the various training periods for a fitness and bodybuilding competitor refer back to chapter 8.)

• Find your motivation. Ask yourself, "Why am I doing this?" More than likely, something inspired you to embark on this journey. Write your motivation down and put it in a place where you will see it often. Review your motivation when you need inspiration or begin to think negatively.

• Make a realistic plan. Much of acquiring the optimal body for a competition depends on timing. For example, losing too much body fat too quickly will cause you to look "stringy," but coming into a competition with too much body fat will not allow your muscularity to show. If this is your first competition, enlist the help of a personal trainer with experience in fitness and bodybuilding preparation.

Exercise 11.1 Mental Game Checklist for Competitive Bodybuilders

The purpose of the checklist is to assist you in examining the mental and physical factors necessary to reach an optimal level of performance. Rate yourself on each of the items at least once every four months, or before each competition. The higher your score the closer you are to your optimal level. If you score 4 or less on certain statements, try to improve in that area before the next competition.

Rating Scale:

1=Strongly disagree	2=Disagree	3=Disagree somewhat
4=Agree somewhat	5=Agree	6=Strongly agree

Training

1. I train in the gym with enthusiasm.

    1   2   3   4   5   6

2. I look forward to my next competition.

    1   2   3   4   5   6

3. I see the next competition as providing me with information about my training progress.

    1   2   3   4   5   6

4. I am very confident in the body that I am creating.

    1   2   3   4   5   6

5. I try to learn something from each training session.

    1   2   3   4   5   6

6. I set goals for each week and month of training.

    1   2   3   4   5   6

7. I set goals for each competition.

    1   2   3   4   5   6

8. I post my goals and review them often.

    1   2   3   4   5   6

9. I am eating proper muscle-building meals.

    1   2   3   4   5   6

10. I am getting at least 7 hours of sleep each night.

    1   2   3   4   5   6

11. My training partner is conducive to my body development.

    1   2   3   4   5   6

12. I have a good social support network.

        1   2   3   4   5   6

Before the Competition

1. I wake up in the morning excited about showing off my hard-earned body.

        1   2   3   4   5   6

2. I enthusiastically anticipate the opportunity to compete in front of spectators and judges.

        1   2   3   4   5   6

3. I look forward to receiving information about my body and training.

        1   2   3   4   5   6

4. I eat a good breakfast.

        1   2   3   4   5   6

5. I remember my goals and I am excited to meet them.

        1   2   3   4   5   6

6. I feel good during the pre-show pump.

        1   2   3   4   5   6

7. I am confident that I will perform well at the competition.

        1   2   3   4   5   6

8. I only speak positively to myself prior to going on stage.

        1   2   3   4   5   6

9. I am relaxed and ready to compete at my very best.

        1   2   3   4   5   6

10. I know my weaknesses and strengths, and plan to highlight my strengths.

        1   2   3   4   5   6

During the Competition

1. I show off my body with zeal and confidence.

        1   2   3   4   5   6

2. I do not let mistakes in my routine discourage me from performing my best.

        1   2   3   4   5   6

3. I am able to show my strengths to the judges and spectators.

        1   2   3   4   5   6

(continued)

Exercise 11.1 *(continued)*

4. I am able to confidently expose the weaknesses of my opponents.

        1   2   3   4   5   6

5. I am in full control of my emotions; neither underaroused nor over-aroused.

        1   2   3   4   5   6

6. During the pose-down, I know what my next move is going to be.

        1   2   3   4   5   6

7. I can recover quickly from surprises during the competition.

        1   2   3   4   5   6

8. I am not overly critical of myself during the competition.

        1   2   3   4   5   6

9. I am excited about getting feedback about my body development.

        1   2   3   4   5   6

10. The crowd excites me, and I can really show off my body.

        1   2   3   4   5   6

After the Competition

1. My performance was my responsibility, no matter the outcome.

        1   2   3   4   5   6

2. I have learned from the judges' feedback.

        1   2   3   4   5   6

3. I already have plans for improvement in the next competition.

        1   2   3   4   5   6

4. The hard work and sacrifices were worth it.

        1   2   3   4   5   6

5. I cannot wait to compete again.

        1   2   3   4   5   6

• Be organized. Preparing for a competition requires attention to a number of factors, including diet (protein, carbs, sodium, and so on), training regimen, strength level, among other things. Therefore, to be successful you must be well organized. To track their progress, most competitive bodybuilders keep logs of their training and eating schedules, and videotape or photograph themselves on a weekly basis.

• Enlist the social support of friends and family. Without a doubt, there will be days when you question yourself, feel like giving up, or are sick and tired of eating chicken and rice. Supportive comments from friends and loved ones can be of great assistance at these times. When you decide to enter a competition, tell your friends and family how they can support you. For example, ask them not to invite you to pizza parties so that you will not feel tempted, ask them to encourage you periodically, or request that they join you on the treadmill occasionally.

Because most people do not understand the intense dedication required in training for a bodybuilding competition, prepare yourself for strange and unsupportive reactions. Some people may not understand why you cannot eat French fries "just once" or why you cannot skip a workout "every once in a while." Moreover, when many people learn about the sport of bodybuilding, they react by asking, "Why would you want to do all that?" When this happens, assess the importance of their support. If they are casual acquaintances, simply let their negative energy bounce off you and forget about it. If they are loved ones or close friends, however, you may want to have a conversation with them about ways to show support, such as those listed above.

• Be patient. This is especially important if this is your first competition. It takes years to build full, mature muscles. You will not look your lifetime best the first time out, nor would you want to.

• Trust your plan. Competitive bodybuilders learn the cutting-up regimen that works best for them through years of trial and error. Nevertheless, many of them still panic in the final weeks before a competition, thinking "I'm too small," "I'm not lean enough," or "I haven't trained hard enough." These thoughts often lead to making drastic changes in diet or training regimen, which may actually diminish their competition performance. It is important to trust your plan; get objective feedback from a trainer or fellow bodybuilder, and avoid making drastic training changes at the last minute.

• Set and celebrate the accomplishment of short-term goals. Twelve weeks is a long time to maintain motivation. Set short-term goals to measure your progress along the way, for example, losing a certain percentage of body fat, successfully performing your posing routine, or using positive self-talk during an entire workout. Then celebrate your accomplishment. Because society typically celebrates accomplishments with food, you will need to be creative about how you will reward your progress. Some examples that do not involve food: getting a massage, going to a movie, or walking around a scenic park or lake for your next cardiovascular workout.

• Stay focused on performance, not outcome. The outcome of a bodybuilding competition is up to the judges. It is out of your control. Therefore, it is important to keep your attention on what you can control: your own performance. Rather than think outcome-focused thoughts, for example,

"Am I going to win?" or "Will I have the best shape in my class?" think about your performance: "Am I following my diet and training plan?" "Am I giving my best effort in the gym?" "Do I feel comfortable performing my posing routine with confidence?"

• Use visualization. Research shows that successful athletes use visualization on a daily basis. Before they begin to prepare for a competition, many bodybuilders construct a mental image of how they want to appear the day of the competition and use that as their motivation. Because your regular training regimen will not include what you do at a bodybuilding competition (posing, for example), you may need to spend extra time learning poses and presenting yourself effectively. Visualization can be of great help with this process. Bodybuilders can visualize their posing routines (while listening to their music), including mandatory poses, and can visualize themselves walking confidently onto the stage.

• Get adequate rest. Without a doubt, preparing for a bodybuilding competition is intense work. In your zeal to be competitive, you may think more about needing to increase your cardiovascular exercise, further restrict calories, and so on, but it is just as important to think about the long term and allow your body to recover. Bodybuilders who try to sprint to the finish will burn out, become injured, or drop out altogether.

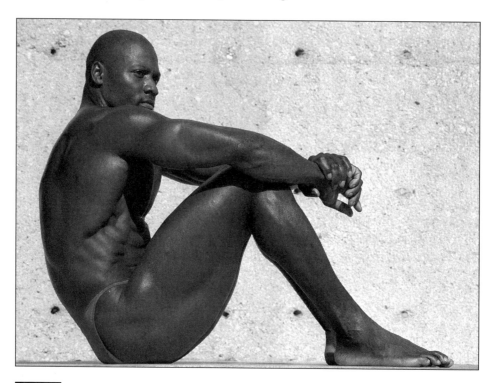

Before competition stay focused on what you can control—your own performance—rather than whether you win or lose.

• Face your fear. Have you ever been scared to do something (for example, speak in front of a large group or pose in a tiny bathing suit) and then, after it was over, wondered what you were so scared about? Think of a competition as a learning opportunity, a setting to discover your strengths and weaknesses from an objective panel of judges. The more competitions you enter, the less fear you will experience about being on stage. Understanding that competitions are essential for long-term development, and that no one event is the ultimate test of your body, is the first step. If you do not challenge yourself, you will not improve. Competitions provide a series of challenges. Moreover, the mental and physical preparation strategies you develop in lower-level competitions will go a long way in helping you create the body you desire, the body of your dreams.

• Stay positive. You will have setbacks during your pre-competition phase. You may become ill, incur an injury, or experience stress in your personal life. Try to learn something from these situations, and then move on. Also, try to find a few positive things from the day that you can think about in the evening before bed. Try to find one positive element from your workout, one from your nutritional habits, and one from the rest of your day.

• Have fun! Bodybuilding competition is serious, but you should still enjoy this process. More than likely, you are doing this for recreation, probably in addition to a full-time job and other responsibilities. Thus, you probably have enough stress in your life. Try to avoid making bodybuilding competitions another one. You probably became a competitive bodybuilder because it sounded like fun. Remember to keep it that way.

During your 12-week pre-competition journey, you will undergo numerous changes. In addition to changes in your appearance, the following factors will drastically change as well: your diet, your training program, the tone of your skin, the amount of body hair you have, the amount of free time in your schedule, and how people react to you.

Diet

Of these factors, diet is probably the most difficult in the pre-competition period. To properly showcase their muscularity, bodybuilders must shed body fat. This requires the manipulation of caloric intake as well as the ratio of protein, carbs, and fats they consume. These dietary changes are often accompanied by feelings of fatigue, irritability, and cravings for restricted foods. If you do not employ effective mental strategies, these feelings can ruin your workouts and may make loved ones avoid being around you.

Oftentimes, merely acknowledging that you feel irritable and talking about it is all you have to do. You may also find thought stopping (see chapter 6) and other cognitive restructuring exercises (see chapters 8 and 10) helpful in switching your focus from what you cannot eat to getting ready for the competition. If, after using these strategies, you find that these feeling are still interfering with your ability to train, some changes to your diet might be warranted. Consult with your trainer or an experienced competitive body-builder to determine the best dietary regimen for your needs.

Training Program

When you step on stage the day of the competition, you want your muscles to appear full and firm. To achieve this look, competitive bodybuilders must often alter their training programs. For example, many bodybuilders per-form more isolation exercises with lighter weights and higher reps before a competition. This type of training is quite different from the earlier muscle-building training, which usually emphasizes compound exercises using heavy weights and fewer reps.

As they make these shifts in training, many bodybuilders irrationally believe that their muscles will shrink because they are no longer lifting heavy weights. Clearly, this can cause them great anxiety, particularly before a competition when they want to be at peak muscular development. As noted above, it is imperative that competitors trust their pre-competition program. Such programs exist because they work.

Skin Tone and Body Hair

Before a competition, most bodybuilders darken their skin and remove body hair so that their muscularity and definition can be seen under the bright stage lights. With the amount of high-quality tanning products available, it is no longer necessary for bodybuilders to damage their skin in the sun or with tanning beds. If this is your first competition, you may want to experiment with a few products before the day of the competition to find the product that gives you the most natural-looking, even-toned appearance. You do not want to step on stage looking orange and streaked!

Removal of body hair may be more of an issue for men, especially those who do not currently shave their legs, chest, or arms. While it is normal for men to shave in many sports (for example, swimming and triathlons), some men feel uncomfortable removing body hair, worrying about comments or looks they might get from loved ones and friends. If you do not usually shave your body, you might want to practice several weeks before the competition to determine how your skin will react. If you break out from a certain shaving technique, it is better to learn that now than to discover it for the first time on the day of the competition. You might want to consult with an experienced competitive bodybuilder for tips on when to shave and special products available.

Free Time

As competition day nears, the amount of time you will need to devote to preparation will increase. In addition to weight training, you may have to increase cardiovascular activity, practice mandatory poses and your posing routine, photograph or film yourself performing your routine, find a suit that shows off your physique, cook more meals each day, and practice your mental skills, among other things. As a result, the amount of time you can devote to other activities will decrease.

Bodybuilders often remark that pre-competition preparation is a 24-hour, seven-day-a-week job. The effort and time required, not to mention the lack of time for everything else, can lead to feelings of frustration and isolation. Supportive friends and family members can offer invaluable assistance at this time. Tell your support network how they can encourage and assist you. For example, your friends could help you stay focused on your goals and encourage you to use your free time for things that lead to bodybuilding success. This could include reading bodybuilding magazines or listening through musical selections for posing music. There will also be times when you need to take a mental and physical break from your strict focus on bodybuilding. A movie or a hike may be just what you need.

Others' Reactions

With each passing week of training and pre-competition preparation, you will begin to take on the look of a competitive bodybuilder. As this happens, people may react to you in a wide variety of ways, including awe, fear, and even disgust. If you are a first-time competitor, you might feel uncomfortable with or puzzled by these reactions. As stated above, before you decide to react, it is important to assess how important these people are in your life. It may actually be helpful to laugh about a negative comment (for example, "That's gross") from a stranger on the street. Laughing it off is certainly more helpful than letting it ruin your attitude or enthusiasm for the sport. On the other hand, it is great to hear positive comments from people in awe of your physique as you walk down the street or beach. You have worked hard and deserve to be noticed.

Competition

Congratulations! You have made it to the week of the competition. Reward yourself for your commitment and discipline. The hard work is behind you. Now all you need to do is get your body and mind ready. Do not think that these last few days are not critical to your performance, however, or that now you can deviate from your preparation program. Now is the time to really step up your confidence and determination for a successful competition. The following are some suggestions that will help you get there.

• Trust your plan. Although your body will continue to change throughout this week, as a result of dietary and water changes (see chapter 4), you will not lose a great deal of body fat, nor will you add pounds of muscle. Trust your hard work over the last several months. Trust your plan. Rather than panic, thinking you did not do enough, trust that you did everything you could. Now is the time to be proud of your accomplishments. There will be plenty of time to evaluate your plan after the competition.

• Mentally and physically practice for competition day. This includes walking out on stage, performing mandatory poses, executing your posing routine, and even standing in a relaxed position. Visualize your performance from beginning to end, using your focus words to stay strong, confident, and intense. Practice physically at least once each day and mentally at least twice each day.

• Make a game plan. Decide what type of tanning products you will use, when you will apply them, and who will help you (choose a reliable and experienced person). The same applies to shaving, hair, and makeup assistance you will need (especially for fitness competitors). Plan what you will eat and drink the day of the competition and pack a cooler to bring with you. Always bring more than you need. You do not want to run out of food and appear "flat" on stage. You also might want to decide what you will bring with you in your gym bag, such as extra copies of posing music, extra tanning products, a towel, body oil, and directions to the competition venue. Finally, especially if you are a first-time competitor, you may want to jot down a warm-up routine before the competition, outlining which exercises you will perform to "pump up," in what order, and when to begin. Consult with an experienced bodybuilder if you are unsure about this.

• Know and understand your opposition. Successful bodybuilders know the physical and mental strengths and weaknesses and the emotional makeup of their opponents in a competition. To exploit another bodybuilder's weaknesses on stage and at the same time display your superior development, you must do your homework. If you have biceps like bowling balls, be sure to show them off beside competitors who have biceps like deflated balloons. Show off your "diamond" calves against opponents who have legs that resemble a world-class marathon runner's. Taking advantage of the physical and mental weaknesses of your opponents is not only helpful but also critical if you are to win the prize.

• Get plenty of rest. At this time, your training will decrease so that your muscles can appear full and strong on stage. During your training time, you may want to perform mental rehearsal or engage in some of the anxiety-reducing strategies described in previous chapters. You want to step on stage feeling energetic and strong, not exhausted and weak.

• Create a competitive attitude that is conducive to successful performance. Bodybuilders go into a competition with different attitudes. Some lack confidence while some are overconfident; some become highly anxious while others remain calm; some need encouragement while others are positively focused on doing their best. The attitudes and emotions are

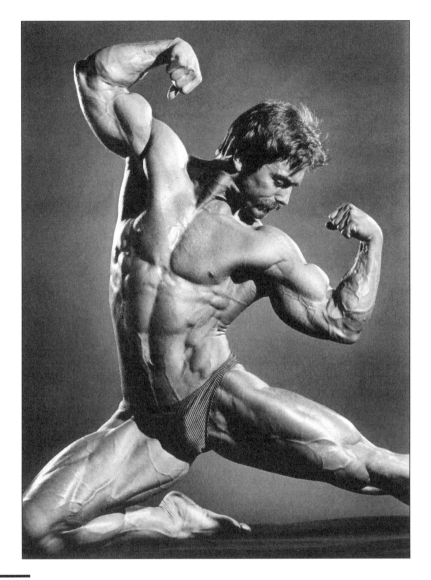

The competition is your opportunity to show off your hard-earned physique.

endless when it comes to the competitive arena. Your job is to develop a competitive attitude that is strong and focused enough to give you the best chance of success.

Remember, unless you are already Mr. or Ms. Olympia, there will always be other bodybuilders who are more muscular, defined, and symmetrical than you are. They may simply have a genetic makeup that allows them to achieve better muscular development and definition. This does not have to prevent you from improving yourself. You can still be a "big fish" in the "big pond" of competitive bodybuilding. You may lose the competition, but if

Competitive Mind-set for Bodybuilding: Neal Hamilton

Neal Hamilton is the 1999 Western Canadian All Natural Bodybuilding Champion. Upon earning his professional card in 1999, Neal finished 11th at the World All Natural Bodybuilding Championships. More than 10 years as a competitive bodybuilder has given Neal these thoughts:

The mental challenges in competitive bodybuilding are in many ways the same challenges that exist in other sports. However, I believe that there are challenges that are unique to bodybuilding. Most important for any bodybuilder is to stay focused 24/7. It can be difficult to stay positive on bad days when everything seems to be going wrong—to keep training with 100 percent effort each and every day. One of my biggest fears is that I will let myself down with inadequate training or diet. But I also know that fear is a good thing because it forces me to give no less than 100 percent in my training and diet. Turning negatives into positives is essential for bodybuilding success.

The most important mental skill for competitive success in my opinion is visualization. When I lay in bed at night, before I go to sleep, I go over the next day's workout, rep by rep, set by set in my own mind. I see myself getting stronger, bigger and more ripped. My brain is like a video recorder—I just have to press play and I know exactly what I need to do. Then when I go to the gym, I lift with focus and intensity. This helps me to remain positive and to believe that I can achieve the goals that I set out to do.

When I am in a competition, I like to try and "psych out" my opponents. One of my favorite things to do is to keep myself covered up back stage in the pump-up room for as long as I can. This keeps them wondering how I look. I just never let myself pay attention to the other competitors back stage. I find that the best way to overcome the "psyching" attempts of the other competitors is to focus on what I have to do to win the show. I will pump-up away from the other bodybuilders and once again, visualize what I have to do on stage come show time. Bodybuilding is about me being on stage in front of hundreds of spectators and the judges. I let my fate be determined by the judges and not the other competitors.

When I am on stage, just prior to the pose-down, my favorite mental strategy is to go to the front of the stage and show the judges my hard-earned body. I do it with total confidence and I try not to worry about anybody else but me. In my head, I am the winner and to be the winner I know that I am going to have to act like a winner on stage. I show off my body in a positive manner that is pleasing to the judges.

you prepare properly and have a positive competitive attitude, you can be confident that you did your very best. Keep your thoughts positive and focused on getting you ready, such as "I feel strong" and "I can't wait to step on stage."

Competition Day

It is finally here, the day you have been working toward. Although many bodybuilders feel relief and excitement on the day of the competition, others feel overwhelming anxiety and begin to doubt themselves. Indeed, it takes great courage to stand nearly naked in front of a panel of strangers while they critique your physique! No matter what their preparation programs, even experienced bodybuilders can feel anxious about competing and performing. After all, competing is not a frequent part of training. Remember, to be successful you will have to have an attitude and the mental awareness that leads to a good performance. The following are some suggestions for achieving a successful competitive experience.

• Bring support. Ask friends and loved ones to come to the prejudging as well as the night competition. Most spectators attend only the evening competition, but you will probably need their encouragement more during the prejudging, when your performance is more critical (the night competition is usually not judged).

• Be confident and positive. You should not be shy and meek during a competition, certainly, but this does not mean that you should present yourself as arrogant or talk badly about other competitors either. Confidence and poor sportsmanship are not the same. Keep your thoughts positive and focused on getting your mind and body ready for the competition. Say the following phrases to yourself: "I am ready," "I look my best," "I feel strong," and "I can't wait to get on stage."

• Be proud of yourself and what you have accomplished. Few people possess the discipline and determination to withstand preparing for a bodybuilding competition. You have trained hundreds of hours for these few moments. Enjoy them!

• Focus on the present. Avoid thoughts like "I should have done more cardiovascular training," or "I didn't load up on enough carbs." Thinking this way will only hurt you, especially during a competition. It will deflate your self-confidence and lead to self-doubt. Instead, keep your mind on what is happening right now. You have worked too hard for this moment to now spoil it with self-doubt. Focus on what you must do to perform your best. Likewise, avoid comparing yourself to your opponents. You have no control over what they do or how they look; you only have control over yourself.

• Manage your anxiety. Use the mental strategies presented throughout this book to keep your anxiety in check. For example, find a quiet place where you can perform complete-breathing exercises, visualize your performance, and engage in positive self-talk. Most bodybuilders try to stay off their feet before they go on stage to avoid fluid build-up in their legs. Doing this will give you a great opportunity to practice your mental skills and prepare yourself to step on stage in an optimal state of arousal.

Presenting Yourself on Stage

The art of presentation in a bodybuilding competition is difficult to learn. Think about it: You are standing nearly nude in front of an audience (including a panel of judges) and you are supposed to appear as if you are having the time of your life! You are obviously going to be filled with anxiety. Regardless of how you feel or what you are thinking about, the way you present yourself to the judges significantly influences your placement. Judges are looking for the whole package: a lean, muscular competitor with confidence and excellent stage presence. You must make yourself stand out, both in intensity and enthusiasm. It is fine to feel nervous, but rather than let your anxiety defeat you, try to turn it into positive energy. The following are some additional suggestions for stage presentation.

• Go for it! Now is not the time to hold back or worry about looking silly. Now is the time to show the judges everything you have. If necessary, find a supportive person in the audience and imagine that you are performing for him or her.

• Exude confidence. You must look like a winner. Self-assurance should be dripping off you like sweat. This includes appearing comfortable, as though you do this every day. Even if you happen to feel different inside, think to yourself, "I am having the time of my life," and "I love this." Competitive bodybuilders often use positive self-talk when a competition gets especially stressful. For example, when an opponent is making a comeback, they think to themselves, "Bring it on. Bring it on."

• Imagine that you are the only person onstage. Once you get on the stage, the only person that matters is you. The number-one sin in competitive bodybuilding is to let another bodybuilder throw you off your strategy by taking away your focus. Your focus should be on your presentation and ways in which you can show the judges that your body is superior to any other competitor. A quick glance at another competitor is all you need to determine your next move.

• Allow your personality to show. In addition to a lean and muscular physique, judges look for that "something special" in a competitor. No, your personality alone will not win the overall title, but it could make a difference if you and a competitor are very close in terms of your physiques. This is called "stage presence," and more often than not, it is the deciding factor in a competition. Be yourself. Show the judges who you are, and have fun.

After the Competition

The competition is over. You have had some ice cream, taken about three showers to scrub off your tanning products, and slept more than you have in months. Competitive bodybuilders typically fill their days after a compe-

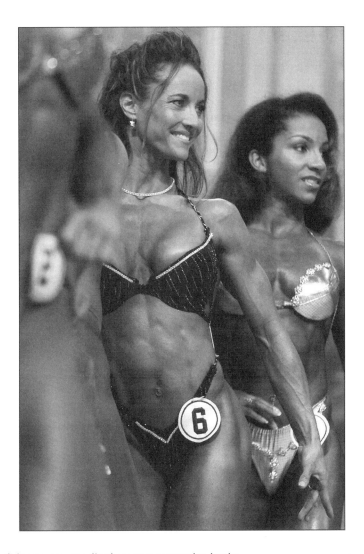

Exude confidence as you display your muscular body.

tition with food (eating all those restricted foods and treats), rest, and time away from the gym. A two- to four- week break away from the gym will not be detrimental to your muscular development in the future. In fact, it will be helpful. For most bodybuilders, this is an enjoyable part of the bodybuilding lifestyle. Some bodybuilders, however, find themselves lost during this time and struggle as they return to their off-season training. The following are some suggestions that will help ease the transition to the off-season.

• Take pride in your accomplishment. Allow yourself to feel the satisfaction associated with setting a goal and then staying determined and focused. No doubt, you experienced challenges and were tempted to give up, but you persisted. Congratulate yourself for your hard work and fortitude.

• Relax and recover. You may be filled with excitement about the sport and your potential after a competition. Nevertheless, avoid all temptation to return to the gym immediately. You have just completed the pre-competition phase consisting of intense training and restrictive dieting, which has put a certain amount of stress on your body. Returning to training too soon can set you up for illness, injury, and burnout. It can also hinder your long-term development. Giving your body ample rest now will allow you to return to the gym refreshed and ready to meet your goals for your next competition.

• Evaluate your plan. Ask yourself the following questions, "What did I do well?" "What would I change or do differently?" Judges and trainers can also provide useful feedback on your training program and competition plan. Remember, however, each opinion you receive is just one person's opinion. There are as many opinions as there are people. In addition, avoid blaming and negative thinking. There is no such thing as failure. The judges' results and your placing at the competition gives you essential feedback that will make you better in the future. If you were disappointed with some aspect of your competition, learn from that experience and try something different during your next competition.

• Allow yourself time for transition. Believe it or not, you may actually miss some aspects of the pre-competition lifestyle. For example, you may find it difficult to lose that lean, competitive look, or you might miss all the structure in your day. You may even struggle to recall what you did with your time before the competition. Merely being aware of this potentially awkward time can be helpful. In addition, give yourself some time to adjust to off-season living. Getting used to such a big change in lifestyle will take some time.

• Transfer your skills. As you reflect on the pre-competitive phase and the presentation period, think about the qualities you learned and perfected: commitment, discipline, patience, fortitude, confidence, and determination. Do not let them sit on the shelf until your next competition. Instead, use them to achieve goals in other areas of your life. Set some long- and short-term goals at work, or make a commitment to improve a relationship that is important to you.

Preparing for and competing in a bodybuilding competition is a long journey, filled with many rewards, sacrifices, and challenges. Given the intense dedication needed to complete this journey, it is no wonder that more bodybuilders talk about competing than actually follow through with their plans. If approached with a positive attitude, a sense of commitment, and an enjoyment of the process, however, this journey can be a wonderful adventure. The mental skills and tips for competition outlined in this chapter enable you to achieve more than you ever imagined.

ENDNOTES

Chapter 1

1. http://www.ifbb.com/

Chapter 2

1. Moore, D. 1993. Body image and eating behavior in adolescents. *Journal of the American College of Nutrition.* 12: 505-62.

2. Fox, K. 1988. The self-esteem complex and youth fitness. *Quest.* 40: 230-46.

3. Rodin, J., L. Silberstein, and R. Striegel-Moore. 1984. Women and weight: A normative discontent. *Nebraska Symposium on Motivation.* 32: 267-307.

4. Wankel, L.M., C.A. Hills, J.C. Hudec, W.K. Mummery, J.M. Sefton, J. Stevenson, and B.G. Whitmarsh. 1994. Self-esteem and body image: Structure, formation, and relationship to health-related behaviours (report submitted to the Canadian Fitness and Lifestyle Research Institute).

5. Vernacchia, R., R. McGuire, and D. Cook. 1992. *Coaching mental excellence: It doesn't matter whether you win or lose.* Cited in J.M. Hogg. 1995. *Mental skills for swim coaches.* Edmonton, Canada: Sport Excel.

6. Waitley, D. 1987. *The psychology of winning.* Chicago: Nightingale-Conant.

7. Goleman, D. 1995. *Emotional intelligence: Why it can matter more than IQ.* New York: Bantam Books.

8. Salovey, P. and J. Mayer. 1997. *Emotional development and emotional intelligence.* New York: Basic Books.

Chapter 3

1. Syer, J. and C. Connolly. 1984. *Sporting Body Sporting Mind.* Cambridge: Cambridge University Press.

2. Kraemer, W.J. 1994. General adaptations to resistance and endurance training programs. In T. Baechle, ed. 1994. *Essentials of strength training and conditioning.* Champaign, Il.: Human Kinetics. 127-44.

3. Kraemer, W.J. 1994. Neuroendocrine responses to resistance exercise. In T. Baechle, ed. 1994. *Essentials of strength training and conditioning.* Champaign, Il.: Human Kinetics. 87-107.

4. Ibid.

5. Incledon, T. and L. Gross. 2000. Cortisol: Bodybuilder's friend or foe? *Muscle and Fitness* (January). 138.

Chapter 4

1. Taylor, W.N. 1985. *Hormonal manipulation.* London: McFarland.

2. Ibid.

3. Ibid.

Chapter 5

1. Kraemer, W.J. 1994. General adaptations to resistance and endurance training programs. In T.R. Baechle, ed. 1995, *Essentials of strength training and conditioning.* Champaign, Il.: Human Kinetics.

2. Baechle, T.R., ed. 1995. *Essentials of strength training and conditioning.* Champaign, Il.: Human Kinetics.

3. Garfield, C.A. and Bennett, H.Z. (1984). *Peak performance: Mental training techniques of the world's greatest athletes.* Los Angeles: Tarcher.

Chapter 6

1. Hogg, J.M. 1995. *Mental skills for swim coaches.* Edmonton, Canada: Sport Excel.
2. Seligman, M.E.P. 1990. *Learned optimism.* New York: Alfred A. Knopf.

Chapter 7

1. Iso-Ahola, S.E. and B. Hatfield. 1986. *Psychology of sports.* Dubuque, Iowa: Wm.C. Brown.
2. Egan, S. 1987. Acute-pain tolerance among athletes. *Canadian Journal of Sport Sciences.* 12, 175-178.
3. Melzack, R. and P. Wall, P. 1988. *The challenge of pain. (3rd ed.)* New York: Basic Books.
4. Goldberg, A.S. 1997. *Sports slump busting.* Champaign, Il.: Human Kinetics.

Chapter 8

1. O'Block, F.R. and F.H. Evans. 1984. Goal setting as a motivational technique. In J.M. Silva and R. S. Weinberg, eds. *Psychological foundations of sport.* Champaign, Il.: Human Kinetics.
2. Orlick, T. 1986. *Psyching for sport.* Champaign, Il.:Human Kinetics.
3. Syer, J. and C. Connolly. 1984. *Sporting Body Sporting Mind.* Cambridge: Cambridge University Press.
4. Ibid.
5. Porter, K. and J. Foster. 1986. *The mental athlete.* New York: Ballantine Books.
6. Wathan, D. 2000. Periodization concepts and applications. In T. R. Baechle, ed. *Essentials of strength training and conditioning.* Champaign, Il: Human Kinetics.
7. Ibid.

Chapter 9

1. Andes, K. 1995. *A woman's book of strength: An empowering guide to total mind/body fitness.* New York: Perigee.
2. Smolak, L., S.K. Muren, and A.E. Ruble. 2000. Female athletes and eating problems: A meta-analysis. *International Journal of Eating Disorders.* 27: 371-80.
3. Ban Breathnach, S. 1998. *Something more: Excavating your authentic self.* New York: Warner Books. 85.
4. Kilbourne, J. 1999. *Deadly persuasion: Why women and girls must fight the addictive power of advertising.* New York: Free Press.

Chapter 10

1. Syer, J. and C. Connolly. 1984. *Sporting body sporting mind.* Cambridge: Cambridge University Press.
2. Ibid.
3. Nideffer, R.N. 1985. *An athlete's guide to mental training.* Champaign, Il.: Human Kinetics.
4. Benson, H. 1975. *The relaxation response.* New York: Avon Books.
5. Benson, H. 1984. *Beyond the relaxation response.* New York: Berkley Books.
6. Gauron, E.F. 1984. *Mental training for peak performance.* Lansing, NY: Sport Science.
7. Hogg, J.M. 1995. *Mental skills for swim coaches.* Edmonton, Canada: Sport Excel.
8. Ibid.
9. Ibid.
10. Syer, J. and C. Connolly. 1984. *Sporting body sporting mind.* Cambridge: Cambridge University Press.

Chapter 11

1. Anshel, M. 1997. *Sport psychology.* Needham Heights, MA.: Allyn & Bacon.

INDEX

Note: The italicized *f* and *t* following page numbers refer to figures and tables, respectively.

ABOUT THE AUTHOR

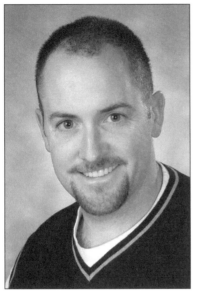

Blair Whitmarsh has the unique background needed to write such a special book. He is a certified strength and conditioning specialist and a member of the National Strength and Conditioning Association. He also holds a PhD with a focus on sport psychology and is a member of the Association for the Advancement of Applied Sport Psychology.

Whitmarsh is consulted by many bodybuilders and strength trainers looking to enhance their training and performance. Whitmarsh is a regular contributor to the popular magazine Muscle and Fitness, and his articles appear in many other related publications. He is also a frequent presenter at conferences, often speaking about the psychological aspects of strength training and bodybuilding.

Whitmarsh is chairman of the department of human kinetics at Trinity Western University in British Columbia. A resident of Langley, British Columbia, Whitmarsh enjoys bodybuilding, running, cycling, swimming, playing tennis, reading, and spending time with his wife, Lorraine, and family.

About the Contributor

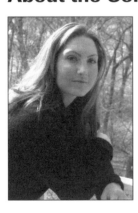

Heidi Paa contributed the chapter on women and bodybuilding, provided much of the material for the chapter on competitive bodybuilding, and served as an expert reviewer on the book. Paa is both a bodybuilder and a counseling psychologist, with a PhD from the University of Nebraska. Her work is published frequently in fitness and bodybuilding magazines. She is now a staff psychologist at the University of Wisconsin in Madison.

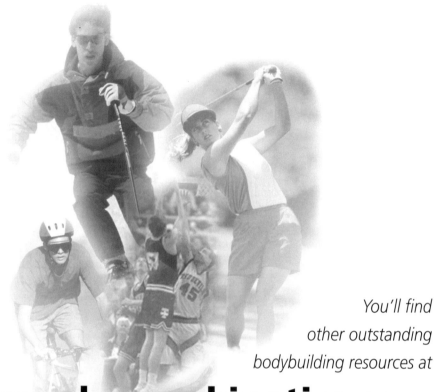